1985

RESTRUCTURING HOSPITAL QUALITY ASSURANCE

THE NEW GUIDE FOR HEALTH CARE PROVIDERS

RESTRUCTURING HOSPITAL QUALITY ASSURANCE

THE NEW GUIDE FOR HEALTH CARE PROVIDERS

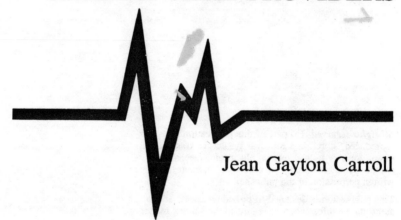

Jean Gayton Carroll

DOW JONES-IRWIN Homewood, Illinois 60430

© DOW JONES-IRWIN, 1984

This publication is designed to provide accurate and
authoritative information in regard to the subject matter
covered. It is sold with the understanding that the
publisher is not engaged in rendering legal, accounting, or
other professional service. If legal advice or other expert
assistance is required, the services of a competent
professional person should be sought.

*From a Declaration of Principles jointly adopted by a Committee
of the American Bar Association and a Committee of Publishers.*

ISBN 0-87094-541-6

Library of Congress Catalog Card No. 84–71132

Printed in the United States of America

1 2 3 4 5 6 7 8 9 0 BC 2 1 0 9 8 7 6 5

Preface

A decade of experience in assisting health care facilities to design and implement their quality assurance, utilization review, and risk management programs has generated some observations about program structure and the perception of quality assurance on the part of hospital trustees, administration, and medical staffs.

Contrary to one of the popular misconceptions, quality assurance is not the screening of medical records and the production of reports. These are simply ways of collecting and reporting data. Quality control and quality assurance are matters of business policy in the health care industry as they are in other industries. Policy cannot be implemented in the absence of appropriate organizational structures. So far the hospital industry in general has overlooked this basic fact and has failed to make adequate organizational provisions for quality assurance.

A large portion of the responsibility for this situation rests with hospital trustees, who, for the most part, have failed to exercise the authority vested in them to provide informed direction to the hospital's efforts to maintain a high quality of patient care. Only with the active support of hospital governing bodies can genuine progress be made in quality assurance.

Jean Gayton Carroll

v

Contents

History and Public Policy Issues

PART ONE

1

The Evaluation of Quality in Health Care Facilities

It is now 10 years since hospitals seeking accreditation by the Joint Commission on Accreditation of Hospitals (JCAH) were first required to develop their own programs for the formal, documented evaluation of the quality of their patient care. During this period the effectiveness of the JCAH quality assurance standards and of hospitals' efforts to comply with them have been under constant and critical evaluation by the health care industry, consumer groups, and the federal government.

Hospital quality assurance as an organizational program has not fulfilled its promise. The entire concept has become mired in evaluation reports, endless committee meetings, and repeated follow-up studies that fail to reveal desired changes. The best efforts of health care professionals to conduct successful hospital quality assurance programs have been frustrated by certain peculiarities of hospital organization structure.

In many hospitals quality assurance activities are poorly organized, largely unsupervised, characterized by the absence of strong central direction, and far less effective than they could be. One outstanding problem is the fragmented nature of the activity.

Despite early JCAH admonitions calling attention to the inter-dependent relationship between utilization review and quality assurance, the quality assurance activities in most hospitals are carried on without reference to related programs, such as malpractice avoidance, utilization management, and reimburse-ment management.

Continual readjustment of review schedules and documenta-tion styles is not going to change this. The only way to deal with the present ineffectual state of hospital quality assurance is through organizational restructuring of the program and of certain related activities.

In analyzing the status of quality assurance activities in Amer-ican hospitals today it is useful to begin with the following issues, each of which has a bearing on developments in the quality assur-ance programs of the future:

- The evaluation of professional performance as influenced by technological advances and the division of labor, and the changing roles of institutions and individuals in the provision of health care services.
- Development of the concept of hospital corporate liability.
- Institutional approaches to the evaluation of health care.
- Legislative developments after 1965.

The Evaluation of Professional Performance

The evaluation of performance is not a new concept. It has been an accepted aspect of industrial life and culture for many centuries. The procedures used to measure performance, however, change from time to time, reflecting changes in technology and organization.

Evaluation and assurance are two different things. In evaluat-ing the quality of a performance or a product, we apply measure-ments related to some criterion or set of criteria. To ensure high quality, we must go beyond that. The mere knowledge of the existence of a problem does not guarantee that it will be resolved—it's only the first step. Quality assurance efforts require organizational structures and procedures to be established, activi-

ties to be prescribed and monitored, and outcomes to be documented and measured. This process calls for an effective authority structure which, for the most part, is nonexistent in health
care facilities.

The health care industry presents some self-imposed handi-
caps to the concept of quality assurance. In place of systematic
objective measurement based on stated criteria, the health care
industry has traditionally relied on the subjective self-assessment
that has always been characteristic of the professional. This
approach implies the absence of a peer group capable of objective
evaluation—a situation that may have prevailed in earlier centuries, but one that certainly has not been the case in the past 60
years, during which time patient care has shifted from the home
to the hospital and other facilities.

Reliance on self-evaluation reflects the idea that professional
performance is related more to art and personal genius than to any
sort of scientific activity that might be duplicated by other practitioners. This approach made sense in the middle ages and would
continue to apply in any field in which effective processes cannot
be precisely defined, analyzed, taught, and reliably duplicated.

However, some of the consequences of sweeping societal
changes during the past century have been reflected in the organization of the health care delivery system. One such change, the
increasing intensity of the division of labor, has had a profound
effect on performance evaluation in the health care delivery
system.

The effects of this development have been obvious in such
fields as manufacturing and distribution for two centuries, but it
took several wars to bring to the health care industry a system
analogous to mass production. From the practices developed on
battlefields during the 19th and 20th centuries there evolved not
only new techniques but more highly structured organizational
forms for the delivery of medical care.

Rapid technological advances, population growth, and the
development of large institutions for health care combined to
necessitate changes in the delivery of health care services. Some
of the tasks once performed by physicians or nurses were delegated to new groups of technicians who were trained in the
performance of highly structured, circumscribed procedures.
These tasks often involved the use of complex equipment that

simplified and routinized the worker's contribution to the job.

This fragmentation of work that formerly was the exclusive province of a relatively small number of individuals who had undergone many years of professional training meant that much of the work was now being performed by new, relatively young persons whose education did not typically include a decade or more of preemployment socialization in the code of the traditional medical professional. The new practitioners tended to be young because their disciplines were new. The nature of their work caused their approach to performance evaluation to be process oriented. They were taught, for example, that their objective was to produce a certain number of accurate test results over a given period of time or for a given number of tests. Whether the test performed was needed or appropriate was not their concern. In many instances they never even saw the patient.

In addition to the growth of the new technical disciplines, the past 25 years have seen an ever-increasing utilization of semi-skilled personnel in health care facilities to assist with certain routine aspects of nursing care under the supervision of professional nurses. An example of the new job classifications that developed during the first 30 years of this century is the nurse's aide. The training of personnel in increasingly routinized, repetitive tasks that could be delegated to them by the professional nurses and technologists came later.

All of these developments in patient care meant that the old ways of evaluating the quality of care were no longer appropriate. In the presence of a heterogeneous population of providers performing a wide variety of services, it was unrealistic to attempt to apply traditional concepts of evaluation that had developed during an era characterized by years of preemployment socialization and scientific training.

The Emergence of the Concept of Hospital Corporate Liability

The traditional image of a medieval refuge for the care of the sick—usually of the indigent sick—is familiar to hospital administrators and professional staff members. Such a facility was typically managed by the members of a religious order that was dedicated to the care of those who had no other place to which to turn in their hour of need. In those days, and for centuries thereafter, the principal activity of any value to the patient consisted of nursing care and emotional support. If the patient required surgical intervention, he might be attended by a physician. These practitioners were usually described as visitors or visiting physicians. They visited the hospital to see their patients, but neither they nor those who operated the facility felt that they owed any accountability to the hospital.

The hospital, in turn, acknowledged no liability for the actions of the visiting physicians and surgeons. Both the hospital and the physician were doing the patient a favor by even attempting to alleviate his condition, and the patient was duly grateful for their ministrations. As recently as the 19th and early 20th centuries, these relationships would probably have been agreed on by the parties as accurately reflecting their roles in the transaction.

It was not until after World War II that the health care industry no longer viewed the hospital as a specialized hotel intended for the housing, feeding, and monitoring of sick people whose physicians had decided that they should be placed in a sheltered environment. In fact, prior to the establishment of university programs in hospital administration, it was not uncommon for lay hospital administrators of the 1930s and 40s to come from the field of hotel management.

For a variety of reasons, including the development of the role of the government as a third-party payer, rising expectations paralleling rising standards of living, and the intensified emphasis on civil rights, hospital patients gradually lost their unquestioning attitude toward hospital services. During the late 1960s laypeople began to examine and evaluate the quality of the care they were receiving. For a long time this evaluative attitude remained focused principally on the salaried employees of the hospital itself, such as nurses, technicians, and ancillary personnel. Eventually, even the physicians came under lay scrutiny.

Until very recently hospitals were not held liable by the courts for the consequences of the actions of medical staff members who were not hospital employees. This attitude was consistent with the old view of the attending physicians as members of an independent professional group whose members merely used the hospital's facilities in the treatment of their patients. While the members of the group organized themselves as a medical staff in order to carry out their organizational functions and responsibilities, the courts, in ruling on malpractice actions, did not hold the hospital itself accountable to the patient for the performance of an individual medical staff member within its precincts.

However, with the precedent established in the landmark Darling case in 1965, the courts have moved slowly but inexorably toward support of the concept of hospital corporate liability for medical staff performance. It has been observed by legal scholars that recent decisions appear to reflect the affirmative duty of a hospital to monitor the quality of care provided by the medical staff.[1]

This trend obliterates the perception of the hospital as hotel. The hospital and its board of trustees cannot escape responsibility for the quality of performance of all those who provide health care services on its premises or under its sponsorship. The inescapable conclusion is that "There is a growing body of law in this country that hospitals have a separate duty running directly from the hospital to the patient to monitor the quality of care rendered within their walls, and, as an element of that duty, to monitor continually the competence of physicians practicing medicine in their institutions."[2]

The surge in the volume of malpractice suits filed against hospitals and medical staff members during the early and middle 1970s has caused the rapid development of risk management as a corporate function, utilizing and relying on systems of constant monitoring of clinical quality.

Institutional Approaches in the United States

Even before the enormous increase in the number of hospital beds that followed World War II, the issue of evaluating physicians' performance was being addressed. One of the earliest proponents of a systematic, objective approach to quality measurement was Dr. Ernest A. Codman, one of the founders of the American College of Surgeons. Codman's 1913 report to the Philadelphia County Medical Society, in which he endorsed the evaluation of a hospital by means of evaluating the end results of its patient care, was a landmark contribution to quality assessment. In Codman's words "every hospital should follow every patient it treats, long enough to determine whether or not the treatment has been successful and then to inquire if not, why not?"[3] In 1913 this was a fairly innovative attitude.

The first convocation of the new American College of Surgeons in November 1913 was another milestone on the road to systematic, organized efforts to improve the quality of patient care in hospitals. In 1914 the college adopted as one of its fellowship requirements that a candidate submit an abstract of at least 50 consecutive major operations that he had performed. This abstract was to contain comprehensive detailed reports on the procedures used, any complications resulting, the elapsed time of the operation, and every aspect of the patient's condition.

The attempts to meet this requirement revealed the generally poor quality of hospital records of the period. As a result the college gave the highest priority to establishing a formal program for the purpose of improving hospital standards, the quality of medical documentation, and the quality of patient care. The plan, established in 1918, was called the Hospital Standardization Program of the American College of Surgeons. Hospitals that met the standards set up by the college received ACS approval and became identified as institutions in which care of the highest quality was provided.

The program was so successful that by 1951 the responsibility of conducting it, which involved hospital surveys taken throughout the country, was a financial burden on the college. Hence in 1952 the college was joined by the American College of Physicians, the American Medical Association, the Canadian Medical Association, and the American Hospital Association to form a successor organization—the Joint Commission on Accreditation of Hospitals (JCAH). Subsequently the American Dental Association joined as a parent organization of the JCAH. At the end of 1958 the Canadian Medical Association withdrew from membership to join the newly formed Canadian Council on Hospital Accreditation.

In April 1953 the JCAH published its first manual of standards for hospital accreditation, which was nine pages long. The standards were divided into two sets: required and contingent. Compliance with the required standards was mandatory for all hospitals seeking accreditation. The contingent standards would be applied to certain hospitals "dependent upon the type, size, degree of departmentalization, and financial resources of a particular hospital." There was no indication in the manual as to how the JCAH planned to identify these hospitals.

Over the next 12 years hospital participation in the survey and accreditation program of the Joint Commission continued to expand rapidly. With a three-year accreditation cycle, the Joint Commission was surveying about 1,100 hospitals a year. The program was financed by the parent organizations for years, but in January of 1964 the JCAH instituted a schedule of charges for the accreditation surveys. During this period the commission continued to emphasize its interest in the maintenance of a high level of quality in patient care as the basis for accreditation. However, it did not introduce any specific techniques for evaluating quality.

Legislative and Regulatory Policies after 1965

One side effect of the Medicare legislation of 1966 was the positioning of the federal government, through the Department of Health, Education and Welfare (HEW), as a major purchaser of hospital services. By virtue of its position, the federal government assumed a new responsibility: the surveillance of the quality of services for which it was financially responsible.

The regulations established to govern implementation of the act provided, among other things, that those hospitals that met the conditions of participation were eligible for Medicare reimbursement. In an effort to make the whole program politically acceptable to the organized medical profession and the hospital industry, the regulations provided that any hospital that was accredited by the Joint Commission would be deemed by the HEW secretary to have met the conditions of participation.

This development obliged the JCAH to review its standards and survey practices critically, and to examine its credibility. With support from the Kellogg Foundation, the JCAH carried out this mandate. This effort culminated in the adoption in 1970 of a new set of standards for the evaluation of hospitals. The new standards, which dealt chiefly with structural criteria, were accompanied by an ongoing program designed to develop more objective and critical surveying techniques.

By 1972, with the federal government established in its role as the primary third-party payer for hospital services, Congress was responding to pressures from many sources demanding revision of the statute and the regulations. Medicare expenditures had risen so rapidly that there were politically popular demands for cost containment. At the same time the philosophy of the Great Society mandated the maintenance of high-quality health care without differentiation among the beneficiaries on the basis of the source of payment. It was politically essential to demonstrate that there was to be no second-class health care for any group of beneficiaries. Furthermore, all segments of the health care industry united to resist any attempts on the part of government to intrude in the relationships among patients and providers.

The compromise solutions that were incorporated in the rules and regulations for implementation of the 1972 Amendments to the Social Security Act appeared, at the time, to be sound and practical. They involved the establishment of two programs through which the hospital industry was to police itself: utilization review and quality assurance.

To remain eligible for participation and reimbursement, a hospital was required to conduct a utilization review—an ongoing review of the use of hospital resources in the care of all federally funded patients. In practice this meant monitoring admissions and length of stay for specified diagnoses and operations. Because cost containment measures were perceived by many as threats to the high quality of hospital care, each participating hospital was required to establish and follow a quality assurance program, including the systematic, objective monitoring of the quality of care given to samples of federally funded patients.

In theory, any hospital that failed to carry out this mandate would be subject to HEW's ultimate sanction—decertification. Decertification would result in ineligibility to receive Medicare and Medicaid reimbursement.

Authority to implement the new regulations and to monitor compliance with the requirements was vested in a new agency within HEW—the Professional Standards Review Organization (PSRO). The PSRO adopted a regional form of organization with local or regional advisory boards representing the providers and the public.

A new program calling for HEW surveys of selected JCAH-accredited hospitals was designed to implement HEW's monitoring role, but this had no impact on the continuing relationship between the industry and the JCAH.

In December 1973 the Joint Commission adopted and published a statement emphasizing the importance of a medical staff quality maintenance program in a hospital's accreditation. The new policy called for retrospective medical audits, continuing education programs, utilization review programs, and application by medical staff credentials committees of medical audit findings in their recommendations for clinical privileges.

During 1974 the JCAH published schedules of required patient care audits. The first schedule, which called for one patient care audit per month for each major clinical service, brought so much protest that the requirement was revised within a few months. The revised schedule differentiated among hospitals on the basis of size with an audit production requirement increasing with the size of the hospital. In March 1975 a new standard entitled "Quality of Professional Services" was published. This document contained detailed requirements for evaluation review and reports.

It gradually became apparent that the JCAH was requiring certain activities in hospitals—specifically in the objective, documented evaluation of performance—that were relatively foreign to most participants in the health care delivery system. As JCAH pressures to comply with the new and increasingly rigorous standards increased, it became obvious that hospital personnel at all levels needed assistance in doing so.

From this need for assistance developed a whole new employment category—the medical record analyst. Medical record analysts were taught to screen records and perform the audits needed to satisfy Joint Commission and PSRO requirements. Their services found a market because of the lack of attention to systematic, objective performance evaluation traditionally demonstrated in the health care field.

For example, in the course of a 1974 survey, of 118 medical schools surveyed, only 24, or 20.3 percent, reported that they offered training in evaluation research. More than 50 percent of these 24 provided no formal instruction in this area other than a single lecture.[4] In a 1980 survey of Chicago-area junior colleges that listed courses in medical record studies leading to the certificate of accredited record technician, it was found that none included any formal instructional material on medical records screening with reference to the review requirements of the JCAH.[5]

During the 1970s the Joint Commission devoted a great deal of effort and expertise to the development of workable techniques for the assessment of the quality of hospital care. During this period the General Accounting Office, after comparing the cost benefits of various systems of hospital evaluation, recommended that the Department of Health and Human Services enter into contracts with the JCAH for surveying hospitals with reference to compliance with the conditions of participation.

However, such arrangements between HEW and the JCAH, a body that was widely perceived as nothing but an arm of the organized health care industry, would have been politically unappealing. HEW settled for maintaining what amounted to a parallel system of survey criteria and procedures, while at the same time trumpeting its resolve to impose the most rigorous and critical monitoring on the Joint Commission's entire accreditation survey process. The relationship between the federal and the voluntary survey and evaluation agencies was in actuality a partnership involving frequent interaction and advisory exchanges.

In the meantime, in the fiscal reimbursement area, the federal government stepped up its efforts to force the hospital industry to curb the rapidly rising increases in costs of hospital care. Cost containment became an objective and a slogan. In an effort to forestall direct government intervention and control of allowable costs, the American Hospital Association devised the "voluntary effort." This approach relied on the voluntary cooperation of individual hospitals in an effort to resist expense escalation in such areas as materials management and salaries. As could have been predicted the effort was so voluntary that it didn't work. Hospital costs rose by approximately 14 percent per year from 1975 to 1980.

Capital costs related to new construction, reconstruction, and equipment acquisition constituted a significant element in the steady rise of health care expenditures throughout the 1960s and

70s. Related debt service and depreciation expense entered into the hospital's Medicare reimbursement accounting equations. Therefore, legislative measures to impose ceilings on such expenditures were devised. With passage of the National Health Planning and Resource Development Act of 1974, hospitals became subject to requirements intended to prevent capital expenditures that were perceived to be unjustified in light of community health care service needs.

This statute gave rise to yet another set of agencies—the health planning agencies at the state level and the community-oriented health systems agencies. These agencies were intended to monitor and evaluate hospital capital proposals involving changes in services or the addition of hospital beds that required expenditures above certain stipulated amounts. Their compliance-enforcement tool is the certificate of need.

Despite the introduction of the programs described, the costs of hospital care that were financed by the Social Security Administration continued to rise relentlessly. A basic flaw in the system was that the SSA was paying for Medicare and Medicaid on a cost-plus basis. Hospitals therefore had no incentive to contain costs.

Clearly, the interests of rational public fiscal policy and responsible allocation of Medicare and Medicaid funding demanded the adoption of some method of regulation that would provide a financial incentive for cost containment. Enactment of the Tax Equity and Fiscal Responsibility Act of 1982 (TEFRA) provided an opportunity for the development of regulations that would, it was hoped, serve to implement the health care cost containment policy.

2

The Impact of TEFRA on the Health Care Delivery System

The impact of the Tax Equity and Fiscal Responsibility Act of 1982 (TEFRA) will be briefly summarized with reference to the following major issues and considerations:

- Financial incentives for the monitoring of quality and utilization.
- Demographic and case mix analysis.
- Hospital productivity in the presence of reduced operating margins.
- Defensive practices in the short term.
- Effects of TEFRA on the industry's structure.

Financial Incentives for the Monitoring of Quality and Utilization

The TEFRA regulations include the following provisions with reference to reimbursement of hospitals for Medicare and Medicaid services:

Beginning with the hospital's first cost-reporting period after October 1, 1983

- The limits applied in calculating reimbursement will apply to total inpatient operating costs, excluding capital related, medical education, and malpractice costs. The limit for the first year is equal to 120 percent of the mean cost per Medicare discharge in each hospital grouping, with hospitals grouped on the basis of number of beds and whether the hospital is located in a standard metropolitan statistical area (SMSA).

- The limits are based on the most recently available Medicare cost data updated to the year immediately preceding the year subject to the expanded limits by the estimated average increase in hospital costs. This historical cost per case is to be increased by a projected inflation factor equal to the hospital "market basket" plus 1 percent.

- Each hospital's limit will be adjusted by a case mix index. For each hospital the Health Care Financing Administration (HCFA) will use diagnosis related groups (DRGs) to develop a case mix index that will increase or decrease the hospital's reimbursement limits. The definition of the hospital's case mix will depend on the composition of its patient population in terms of DRGs.

- An incentive target rate will be established for each hospital to control increases in costs per Medicare case for a three-year period. The target rate will be based on allowable costs per Medicare discharge for the preceding reporting period plus an inflation adjustment plus 1 percent.

- A hospital with an operating cost per Medicare discharge below its target amount will be paid its reported cost plus 50 percent of the difference between the reported cost and the target cost, with the bonus not to exceed 5 percent of the target amount.

- A hospital with an operating cost per Medicare discharge that exceeds its target amount will be paid 25 percent of the excess cost in each of the first two reporting periods and none of the excess cost in the third period.

In order to implement these requirements, the Health Care Financing Administration adopted a categorization tool called the major diagnostic category (MDC). Twenty three MDCs have been defined and organized in terms of the usual classification by systems. Each MDC, in turn, is broken down into several diagnosis related groups (DRGs). In all there are 467 DRGs. One additional DRG is defined as an "unrelated operating room procedure to a given MDC."

In theory, any hospital admission or outpatient visit can be defined in terms of one of the DRGs for purposes of reimbursement. The system was designed for application to federally funded hospital care, but other third-party payers are exploring its usefulness for purposes of claim evaluation. The Veterans Administration, although all of its patients are federally funded, is in the process of evaluating the system for application in its hospitals. They have suggested a target application date of 1985.

For reporting years that begin on and after October 1, 1983, hospitals will be reimbursed on the basis of case mix defined in terms of DRGs. Each DRG carries with it an assigned reimbursement amount. Prospective pricing will be phased in over a four-year period, with the payment formula changed each year. In the first year, payment for each Medicare patient will be 75 percent of the hospital-specific cost per case amount plus 25 percent of the regional average price for the assigned DRG. By the fourth year, payment will be based on the urban or rural national average price for the assigned DRG, adjusted for area wage differences. For Medicare accounting purposes, a patient is defined in terms of his primary discharge diagnosis or surgical operation and any co-existing complicating conditions. The hospital will be reimbursed on the basis of this definition. Several observations proceed from this fact.

First, it is essential for reimbursement purposes that diagnoses and treatments be recorded with as much accuracy and precision as possible. When a diagnosis or operative procedure is recorded in terms that are not consistent with one of the DRGs, it will be defined as an invalid identifier and reimbursement will be denied.

Second, the use of the DRG concept in determining the hospital's case mix and the allowable amounts of reimbursement puts a monetary premium on excellence in hospital care. A hospital may no longer claim added costs that are related to excessive lengths of stay reflecting the occurrence of complications resulting from inadequate care.

Third, there is potential for abuse of the DRG system. When the application of nomenclature determines the allocation of reimbursement, the temptation exists to overstate the seriousness of patients' conditions. Another possible abuse might be the "churning" of certain Medicare patients—repeated short admissions for the same diagnosis. The system provides an incentive for this abuse by granting flat rate reimbursments for each admission on the basis of the diagnosis.

Compliance with the HCFA regulations will be monitored and documented by statewide Peer Review Organizations (PROs), which will replace the Professional Standards Review Organizations (PSROs). HCFA plans to have the PROs designated and in operation by October 1, 1984. Each state and the District of Columbia will have a PRO.

Present plans state that each PRO is responsible for conducting utilization review on all federally funded admissions in its state. Five percent of all federally funded admissions are to be reviewed for compliance with the relevant indications for admission. A hospital with an admission denial rate in excess of 2.5 percent of total admissions will be required to submit to a 100 percent admission screening.

The PRO may subcontract with other organizations to perform part or all of the review work. However, it is subject to specific restrictions to prevent subcontracting with organizations that might have a conflict of interest. While it cannot delegate utilization review, the PRO will be permitted to delegate quality assurance review or patient care review to hospitals that can demonstrate competence.

In brief, HCFA's aims are expressed as

- Reduction in unnecessary hospital readmissions due to inadequate care.
- Ensuring the avoidance of underutilization.
- Reduction in avoidable deaths.
- Reduction in unnecessary surgery.
- Reduction in postoperative complications.

Demographic Analysis and Case Mix Analysis

Adoption of the regulations for the implementation of TEFRA has finally provided some compelling incentives for hospitals to evaluate the quality of care and the utilization of resources in patient care. Elimination of the cost-plus basis for reimbursement means that hospitals must scrutinize the rationale for diagnostic studies and treatments far more rigorously than they have in the recent past.

Because the hospital's allocated Medicare budget is largely dependent on its forecasted case mix, new emphasis will be placed on the need for detailed research in the demographic characteristics of the hospital's patient population and of its service area. In addition hospitals will be forced to analyze and evaluate medical staff admission activities and utilization profiles with care. Clear-cut hospital and medical staff policies regarding appropriate cost-effective utilization of the hospital's resources will have to be developed. In the course of these developmental efforts, the administration and medical staff should make use of the expertise and input of the hospital's financial officers and planning staff.

The single most productive source of data on patient origins, patient demographic characteristics, case mix, and physician admission and utilization profiles is the completed medical record. The demands made by the prospective payment system will force hospital financial divisions to take a greater interest in the quality of data found in the medical record. In addition medical record data will have to become readily accessible to the financial staff. The requirements of a sophisticated case mix analysis for administrative decision making will necessitate a closer link between the medical record department and the financial division than has existed in the past.

Perceptions as to the quality of medical record data vary depending on the viewer's personal experience, but there is general agreement that the quality and accuracy of such data are below acceptable standards. In the course of an ongoing survey conducted by the author in 1980 and 81 of over 1,000 charts in 17 hospitals, it was found that the primary discharge diagnosis was inaccurately or incompletely recorded on the face sheet by the attending physician in 33 percent of the cases. It is submitted that many hospitals in this country do not have reliable information concerning their case mixes and demographics.

Because of the crucial effect of data quality and accessibility on claims processing and case mix management, it is becoming

increasingly common to incorporate the medical record department in the hospital's financial structure. Directors of medical
record departments in hospitals that have made this organizational
change report favorably upon the results.

Under this new organization structure, the director of medical
records reports to the vice president for finance or to the chief
financial officer. In a typical example, the task of grouping
discharge data into DRGs is performed in the medical record
department. In a recent poll, it was found that all of the hospitals
that have placed the medical record department in the financial
organization are using microcomputers and commercially developed software for the purpose of grouping discharge data.

Hospital Productivity

For over a generation it has been customary, and often
required by local health department regulations, to staff the nursing and ancillary services of hospitals at all times so as to be
prepared for peak work loads. This statement, in the present
context, is not intended as an argument for the split shift.
However, there is no doubt that the emergency preparedness
philosophy of hospital management has contributed to a certain
degree of overstaffing.

The variation in staffing ratios between investor-owned and
not-for-profit hospitals shows that there is a degree of slack in the
system. In 1982 investor-owned hospitals reported averages of 2.7
full-time employees per adjusted occupied bed, while not-for-
profit hospitals reported an average of 3.45 full-time employees
per adjusted occupied bed. While the relative severity of patients'
conditions was not accounted for in the survey data, the degree of
variation is suggestive of management differences.

Other institutional factors are at work as well fostering a
reluctance to carry out mass layoffs of trained personnel who
might be difficult to rehire or replace on short notice. Market
competition and what is perceived as sound industrial relations
policy work to encourage a certain amount of overstaffing. Therefore, even during periods of low occupancy, nursing services and
other hospital departments tend to "store" valued personnel for
the day when occupancy may rise and additional employees may
be needed.

During 1983 the health care component of the consumer price index (CPI) rose at an estimated rate of 17 percent—approximately five times as much as the CPI itself. A major portion of this rise was attributable to hospital room charges and "other hospital and medical care services," which is based largely on charges for ancillary services. The portion attributable to physicians' services rose by less than 4 percent.

The obvious need to increase productivity will inevitably bring about the use of more sophisticated techniques of analysis. The functional and organizational analyses that must be performed in evaluating the quality of patient care will also provide data for use in the evaluation of productivity.

Since the possibility of overstaffing can exist only in services and departments that a hospital maintains in its organization, hospitals will now review their service mixes in order to eliminate those services that are not cost-effective. Other organizations are already showing their willingness to take up the slack by providing many services on an outpatient basis that cannot be cost-effective in the inpatient setting.

Defensive Practices in the Short Run

Cost Shifting

While the direct impact of the TEFRA-induced changes will fall on Medicare services, the other third-party payers are showing increasingly strong and overt resistance to cost shifting. The term *cost shifting* is applied to a hospital's practice of making up for the losses it incurs in caring for Medicare and Medicaid patients by adding equivalent amounts to its routine charges for services rendered to nonfederally funded patients. In the past cost shifting usually represented the only way in which hospitals could afford to carry their Medicare and Medicaid patients. This avenue of relief is rapidly disappearing with the new militance of the private insurers.

Selective Admission Policies

The federally funded patient is going to become financially unattractive to traditional hospitals. At the same time the old Hill-

Burton hospitals that were built during the 1950s and early 60s are becoming obsolete. Under the terms of the Hill-Burton construction grants, these hospitals were required to provide varying amounts of free care and to accept federally funded patients. Many of the Hill-Burton hospitals are being replaced by new facilities that are financed through private sources of capital and thus will not be subject to the same case mix requirements as their predecessors.

The first 36 to 48 hours of a patient's stay associated with diagnostic studies, usually serve to generate more revenue for the hospital than does any other interval during a hospitalization, with the exception of the day on which a surgical procedure is performed. Therefore, under a system of prospective payment based on a DRG-defined case mix, it will be to the advantage of hospitals to limit lengths of stay.

It will become increasingly important for hospital financial officers to identify those factors that generate excessive lengths of stay. It has been determined that the nonmedical factors, such as ancillary services, that account for only a small part of excessive stays and are actually found in patients whose admissions probably would not have been justified by preadmission screening. In other words, it is the issue of the appropriateness of the admission itself that is crucial in the evaluation of utilization.

Due in part to these developments, many hospitals will begin to exercise a higher degree of selectivity in admissions than they have in the past. It is likely that the new criteria for admission will be implemented subtly in conjunction with the ongoing monitoring and evaluation of the practice patterns of medical staff members. In other words, new screening criteria will be applied to the members of the medical staff. Thus they will be under pressure to divert financially marginal patients from the inpatient hospital and toward other providers. While the predicted surplus of physicians in the next decade may strengthen the bargaining position of the hospitals vis-à-vis the medical staff, it may also increase the number of patients treated in the physician's office.

Manipulation of Admission and Discharge

The Health Care Financing Administration has expressed its concern that some hospitals may adopt a strategy of repeated short-stay admissions for Medicare patients. By following this pattern of utilization, a hospital could increase its number of admissions and discharges thereby increasing its number of reimbursable claims. Since Medicare claims will be paid on the basis of diagnosis or procedure, without reference to the length of stay, it would be to a hospital's advantage to admit and discharge Medicare patients as rapidly and as often as is feasible. An additional HCFA concern is the temptation to permit unjustified admissions.

The most effective way for a hospital to demonstrate that it is not engaging in such practices is to show that it has a rigorous quality and utilization monitoring program coupled with a strong system of guidance and corrective measures. In this way it may retain its delegated quality review privilege.

Effects of TEFRA on Industry Structure

Alternative Providers

An intensified review of the utilization of resources will have an effect in determining not only the case mix but even the site at which patient care is provided. Due to the constraints imposed by a relatively fixed budgetary allocation, Medicare fiscal intermediaries and other third-party payers, many of whom write Medicare supplemental coverage, will search for lower-cost alternatives to traditional inpatient care. Their critical reviews and rejections of claims will force the utilization of ambulatory care providers, home health care services, and hospice programs.

The utilization of alternative providers of patient care had been supported by the expanding field of health maintenance organizations (HMOs) for a number of years prior to TEFRA's enactment. The HMO-generated pressure coupled with the Medicare-generated pressure is bound to result in an increasing demand for services provided in alternative settings.

In response to such institutional constraints as these, hospitals are already restructuring and repositioning themselves so as to be able to deliver services by means of alternatives to traditional inpatient care. As a result of this trend, an increasing proportion of health care services will be delivered through such organizations as ambulatory care facilities, including emergicenters and surgicenters, home nursing agencies, and hospices.

Changes in Size and Number of Hospitals

Because of the high fixed costs and peak-load staffing that are characteristic of small hospitals, economic pressures are effectively squeezing many small hospitals out of the market. Many of them will be acquired by or merge with other institutions during the next decade, continuing a trend that has been documented since 1972. Since 1972 the number of hospitals with 400 or more beds has increased by 30.4 percent, while the total number of short-term general hospitals has remained stable.

Another factor that will have an impact on case mix management is the well-documented trend toward mergers. This trend will result in a reduction in the number of hospitals, with a far higher proportion of them having 400 or more beds than has been the case in the past. Such facilities, many of which will be privately financed and either will belong to or will be operated by investor-owned organizations and systems, will be the beneficiaries of sophisticated professional management. Their financial and competitive positions should be far stronger than those of the smaller, older hospitals that they will replace.

Emergence of a Two-Tiered Delivery System

One possible result of the application of funding and admission criteria could conceivably be the emergence of a two-tiered system of health care with some or many federally funded patients effectively denied access to high-quality inpatient care. The predictable government response to this possibility could take the form of increasingly stringent regulatory requirements for the assessment and maintenance of high-quality care in the facilities of alternative providers. Medicare coverage of services provided through the alternative delivery system would serve to justify the imposition of quality and utilization monitoring measures similar to those now in effect in inpatient settings.

It should be noted that both the JCAH accreditation standards and the federal conditions of participation in the Medicare program prohibit discrimination in hospital admissions on the basis of the source of the patient's funding. However, covert discriminatory policies related to the source of payment are difficult to identify.

One result of prospective payment may be the rationing of medical and hospital services. Expensive services that are available in the hospital may be withheld from certain patients, such as the terminally ill. The development of this type of philosophy with its need for sophisticated decision making will place new strains on the hospitals' quality monitoring systems. The loose organizational structure of present quality assurance programs will prevent them from dealing effectively with rationing problems. This absence of clear medical policies coupled with some perceived economic need for rationing could result in a number of undesirable outcomes. One might be the existence within any one hospital of a wide range of individual sets of subjective, implicit criteria for making life and death selection choices. Another would certainly be the development of an ongoing struggle between the hospital's financial organization and its medical staff.

Preferred Provider Organizations

As an independent or hospital-linked corporation, physicians on a hospital's medical staff can enter into service contracts with self-insured employers and with insurance companies. The corporation, called a preferred provider organization (PPO), agrees to provide office services and in-hospital medical care to the plan's beneficiaries and their dependents at preestablished discounted rates. The payer or plan then provides financial incentives to the beneficiaries to use the services of the PPO. To the extent that groups of medical staff members organize as PPOs and contract with purchasers of health care services, they can serve as generators of nonfederally funded admissions to their hospitals.

The hospital's incentive is the hope of stabilizing its census at an acceptable level and of maximizing occupancy rates of nonfederally funded patients. However, a significant disadvantage to the hospital is that in cases where the PPO includes in its membership the hospital's entire medical staff, there is no way to avoid the possibility of including the physician with inefficient practice patterns that generate excessive costs and thus reduce the hospital's margin.

The banding together of physicians in PPOs means that they

are positioning themselves to compete with the hospital in providing many types of ambulatory care. Technological advances, particularly in such fields as anesthesia and surgery, are making it possible for physicians to perform procedures in their offices or, for example, in freeStanding surgicenters that only a decade ago would have required an admission to the hospital. These technological changes coupled with the increasing economic sophistication shown by physician groups and their professional managers will serve to strengthen the competitive position of the physician vis-à-vis the hospital. Physicians working in their offices or in freestanding ambulatory care facilities will be in a position to offer strong competition to conventional hospitals.

As the volume of services provided in settings other than hospitals increases, with third-party payers providing coverage, pressures for the development of formal quality assurance programs in such settings will inevitably increase.

Physicians' offices are not subject to any sort of systematic, documented quality assurance monitoring or review. Nonhospital ambulatory care facilities can voluntarily apply for evaluation and accreditation to either the Joint Commission on Accreditation of Hospitals or the Accreditation Association for Ambulatory Health Care and must, as a condition of accreditation by either body, maintain acceptable quality assurance programs. However, there is presently no compelling financial incentive, like the old HEW "deemed status," encouraging freestanding ambulatory care facilities to seek accreditation.

One issue that is certain to arise in connection with third-party payer efforts to ensure acceptable quality levels in freestanding alternative facilities is the requirement that a facility either have a transfer agreement with an accredited hospital or that its staff members have admitting privileges at an accredited hospital.

While technological advances offer the physician a bargaining chip in his competitive relationship with the hospital, the existence of a rigorous quality assurance–risk control system can be used to support the hospital's claim that it is the preferred site for the provision of services that could be performed in either setting. Hospitals may, as a competitive tactic, begin to emphasize the high quality of their services in future marketing activities, as certain domestic automakers are currently doing. The advantages of quality assurance monitoring could serve as one way of differentiating among the products and thus may become an effective marketing tool.

Utilization Projections

At present it is almost impossible to develop realistic projections of inpatient utilization for the years 1990 and beyond. This is due to the fact that the full impact of TEFRA and the prospective payment system cannot yet be measured. However, it is safe to predict that the Social Security Administration's interest in utilization and quality of care will not diminish, because the size of the Medicare constituency is not going to diminish.

On the basis of the "most likely" population projections from the Statistical Abstract of the United States, 1982–1983, table 4, it is projected that the population aged 65 and over will increase from 26,833,000 in 1982 to 31,799,000 in 1990 and to 35,035,000 by the year 2000. This represents an increase of 30 percent from 1982 to 2000. By the year 2000, the 65-and-over age group is expected to account for 13.9 percent of the total population.

It is estimated, on the basis of data published by the American Hospital Association in its Monitrend Reports, that the 65-and-over group accounts for 41 percent of hospital inpatient days. The current national standard for beds needed is 4 per 1,000 population. At an 85 percent hospital occupancy rate, that standard would be met at an annual utilization rate of 1,220 patient days per 1,000 population. Assume that by 2000 the national standard for hospital beds needed has been reduced to 3.5 per 1,000 population. At an 85 percent occupancy rate, annual patient days would be 1,100 per 1,000. With the population projected to be 259,000,000, annual patient days would be in the neighborhood of 285,000,000. If it is assumed that 45 percent of all patient days will be attributable to the 65-and-over age group, they will account for approximately 128,250,000 patient days annually.

Despite the anticipated reduction in admission rates and lengths of stay due to the effects of the prospective payment system, it is unlikely that overall utilization rates in the 65-and-over age group can be significantly reduced. There is a strong possibility that any reduction in the hospital admission rate may be at least partially offset by an increase in the average length of stay. This would occur if an increasingly high proportion of admissions were associated with the most severe illnesses.

Given the anticipated restrictions on inpatient admissions, it is projected that the volume of visits to hospital outpatient departments and to alternative facilities will continue to rise. In 1982 there were an estimated 248,000,000 visits to hospital emergency and outpatient departments. A conservative projection for the year 2000 is 278,000,000 visits to all types of ambulatory care facilities.

It is projected that by 1990 the segment of the population aged 65 and over will have increased by 18.5 percent over the 1982 level. The increase in the size of this age group from 1982 to the year 2000 is expected to be 30.5 percent, increasing from 11.5 percent to 13.5 percent of the total population. This is one of two groups whose members would be directly affected by the emergence of a two-tiered delivery system, the other being those eligible for Medicaid.

**Quality Assurance
Programs and
Methodology**

PART TWO

3

Organization Structure and Accountability

The Effects of the Present Organizational Structure

In the 10 years during which hospitals have been developing and revising their quality assurance and utilization review plans and programs to satisfy approval and regulatory requirements, corporate direction of quality assurance activities has been hampered by the traditional self-governing structure of hospital medical staffs.

In failing to acknowledge their responsibilities for the maintenance of high quality in patient care and to exercise their authority with respect to hospital governance, hospital governing bodies, by and large, have provided little effective support to quality assurance programs.

The predictable result is the costly and ineffective character of quality assurance activity typically found in many hospitals today.

A list of the faults commonly found in hospital quality assurance programs would include the following observations:

1. There is no identifiable central body that is responsible for and authorized to direct hospitalwide quality assurance activities.

2. Quality monitoring and control responsibilities and duties are fragmented throughout the organization.

3. There is little or no communication with respect to review plans, study findings, or corrective measures among the many organizational units. This is particularly apparent in the case of the medical staff, which typically fails to share quality monitoring findings with other organizational units.

4. There is no clear assignment of authority for the implementation of corrective actions at any level of the structure or within the various organizational units.

5. Much of what passes for quality review is unreliable because it does not involve the application of preestablished, clearly formulated criteria; objective evaluation techniques; or adequate sampling methods.

Structural Needs and Solutions

No matter how elegantly drafted nor how lofty the intentions of its proponents, a program for the assurance of high quality cannot survive and function effectively unless it rests on a base of acknowledged authority. The major source of weakness in hospital quality assurance programs is the tension that exists in the relationships among the governing body, the administration, and the medical staff. The formulation and implementation of the hospital's quality assurance program was intended to be a joint effort among these three bodies. However, in this process it is necessary to overcome the following four major obstacles:

1. The boards of trustees of many not-for-profit hospitals perceive the quality of professional performance as being the responsibility of the medical staff alone.

2. Health care professionals, physicians and nonphysicians, have traditionally tended to perceive formal departmental or service performance evaluation as a punitive exercise.

3. Hospital administrators subscribe to the quality assurance philosophy but resist taking definitive action because they are

unsure of their authority and fearful of antagonizing health
care professionals.

4. The inappropriate use of hospital personnel in implementing
    the quality assurance program contributes to technical diffi-
    culties and excessive program expense.

The Role of the Hospital Governing Body

In the voluntary hospital systems of the United States today,
there are at least two kinds of hospital governing bodies. One is
the board of directors of an investor-owned system, which may
own one or more facilities and may manage others. Since this
board is oriented toward protecting the system's assets and
generating profits, it takes a strong interest in maintaining the
quality of the organization's product—health care services. The
boards of investor-owned systems are strongly aware of the
connection between poor quality and malpractice exposure. Their
support of administrative efforts to contain the latter shows their
interest in preventive quality monitoring.

Another type of governing body is one commonly overseeing
the operations of the not-for-profit hospital, whether it is a single
facility or a member of a multifacility not-for-profit system. This
board of trustees has its origins in the honorable and unique tradi-
tion of American voluntarism. Many of the attitudes of its
members are reminiscent of those that might have been expressed
by their grandparents when they served on the boards of the same
institutions.

Those board members perceived themselves as individuals
who had been invited to serve the hospital in raising funds and in
mobilizing other community leaders in an effort to bring hospital
care to the needy. Other responsibilities included the maintenance
of links to local officials and bankers whose assistance in connection with building and rehabilitation programs would be valuable.
They represented the best elements of the community in the
hospital's governance, and they represented the hospital to the rest
of the community. The hospital was one of their favorite charities.
Their motives were philanthropic, and election to the board of
trustees was viewed as acknowledgement of community leadership
and personal achievement.

Far from the minds of these trustees was any notion of investigating the quality of patient care that was provided in the hospital. Such behavior, which was seen as interference in the activities of dedicated, learned professionals, was inconsistent with the role of the trustee. Furthermore, such interference would not have been tolerated by the health care professionals who staffed the hospital.

Until the past decade not even the threat of malpractice exposure could have had much effect on the trustees of the not-for-profit hospital. Unless the conditions of agency and respondeat superior could be conclusively shown by a plaintiff's attorney, the hospital itself was not held liable for damage to a patient that was attributable to the actions of a medical staff member. As mentioned earlier, this has changed. With the development of the concept of hospital corporate liability, the trend is in the direction of holding the hospital responsible for actually and substantively monitoring the quality of patient care and for taking needed corrective action.

Despite this broadly publicized development, evidence suggests that the traditional, philanthropy-oriented trustees of the not-for-profit hospital still fail to take appropriate concrete measures to establish and implement rigorous systems for evaluating the quality of clinical care and to support needed corrective measures. The hospital's administration and medical staff are accountable to the governing body, and the governing body is accountable to the community and to society. In other words, one of the governing body's basic responsibilities is its representation of the consumer of health care services. Too many of its members seem to overlook this aspect of governing body accountability. This interpretation of the responsibility of the governing body is reflected in the recent opinions dealing with hospital corporate liability.

Available evidence suggests that even today many hospital trustees feel that as laypersons they would be out of place in directing the review of professional activity. This attitude persists despite the development of the hospital corporate liability concept that was outlined earlier. The governing body that declines to take an active interest in the hospital's quality assurance activities and to deal effectively with the issue of quality control and malpractice exposure is disregarding its responsibility to protect the hospital's financial base and to contain the cost of care. In the face of the reduced operating margins resulting from the effects of prospective payment as well as accelerating competition for the health care dollar, the hospital cannot afford trustee failure in this area.

The absence of a functioning supervisory structure supported by rewards and sanctions has already contributed to malpractice exposure. In addition, under the constraints of prospective payment, which demand precise, accurate and timely documentation of patient care as well as assurance of its appropriateness, the absence of effective controls will result in the denial or reduction of Medicare claims. Therefore, the effectiveness of the hospital's quality assurance, utilization control, and risk control programs is a matter of vital importance to the financial health of the organization.

The fragmentation that presently characterizes quality assurance activities in so many hospitals prohibits the development of adequate authority at any level to implement the true objectives of the program. Quality assurance must be defined as a department.

Since the authority to carry out an organization's activities is defined and explicated through the corporate bylaws, the necessary changes in hospital structure must first be addressed by revising these bylaws. In order to make the organizational provisions necessary to establish a strong quality assurance program, it is essential that the board place responsibility for quality assurance squarely within the hospital's administrative structure through bylaw provisions.

The following steps comprise one way to accomplish the necessary organizational changes:

- Place the responsibility for quality assurance, risk control, and utilization control, including case mix management, in a standing committee within the board of trustees. Identify this group as the committee on standards.
- Set up an office of hospitalwide quality assurance, risk control, and utilization control under the direction of an individual who occupies a position at the vice presidential level and who reports directly to the chief executive officer. Identify this office as the office of standards.
- Schedule quarterly meetings of the committee on standards to

review written reports submitted by the vice president–director of standards.

- Make the budgetary provisions necessary to support the operations of the office of standards.

The time has come to stop thinking of quality assurance as an activity to be carried on by committees, whether of governing body or medical staff, without benefit of a clearly defined place in the organization's operating structure. The issues are sufficiently complex and crucial to the hospital's financial health to warrant organizational recognition.

The Role of the Professional Staff

A major source of confusion concerning the role or roles of the professional and clinical personnel in a hospital is that there are two principal groups of health care professionals functioning within two different organizational structures. One group is the medical staff, which, in a voluntary hospital, forms its own committee organization and reports directly to the governing body through its executive committee. The other large group consists of the nursing service and the ancillary services, which report to the hospital's administration.

The self-governing status of the medical staff is a product of the original relationship between the physician and the hospital— long before the development of the concept of hospital corporate liability and its implications. This status influences the issue of medical staff accountability to the governing body, which is the relationship to be implemented by the hospital's quality assurance program. If this relationship is not acknowledged or not clearly understood by the medical staff, there can be little hope of strong medical staff support of quality assurance, risk control, and utilization control activities.

In one series of surveys conducted in connection with seminars for medical staff members, it was found that 88 percent of the participating physicians believed that the medical staff's executive committee in a hospital is responsible to the organized medical staff rather than to the governing body.[6] This misconception of the essentials of an effective hospital organizational structure contributes to the failure to implement quality assurance programs.

Since the inception of the Joint Commission's efforts to impose effective quality monitoring requirements on hospitals through its accreditation standards, medical staffs have sought to protect themselves from what they perceived to be uninformed, unjustified, and sometimes punitive probing by the agents of hospital administration. Where this perception exists, it interferes with and can destroy any efforts to implement a sound quality assurance program.

Note that the present examination of medical staff structure and function does not address the government hospital with its fully salaried medical staff and clearly defined departmental organization. Rather, it addresses the so-called voluntary hospital in which few, if any, of the attending physicians—those who do not head such hospital-based services or departments as radiology, pathology, respiratory services, and physical medicine—are hospital employees. Most American hospitals fall into this category. The attending physicians, dentists, and others who see patients in the hospital are typically self-employed practitioners or members of group practices. As appointees of the governing body, they acknowledge their obligation to abide by the hospital's policies, but there is no employee relationship.

The typical medical staff, which is composed of self-employed practitioners, has no supervisory structure. In order to carry out their responsibilities in such matters as the review of antibiotic and blood utilization, surgical practice, resource utilization, quality assessment, medical record processing, and the review of the credentials of applicants for staff appointment or reappointment, the medical staff members organize committees. The number of committees varies with the size and complexity of the hospital. Small medical staffs often meet to carry out these functions as a whole—a perfectly appropriate arrangement for some hospitals. The chairmen of the committees comprise the medical staff executive committee, which reports to the governing body.

To a certain extent, professional performance is reviewed and evaluated through these committees. The medical staff's quality assurance committee typically receives and reviews reports dealing with problem areas. However, given the nature of the association and the fact that staff members must work together and rely to a great extent on referrals, it is extremely difficult for any quality assurance committee chairman to initiate or recommend a measure that might have derogatory or punitive connotations. Chairmanship of the quality assurance committee is usually viewed as a thankless job and is accepted only in the spirit of good citizenship. After all, the most effective measure available to the staff through its credentials committee and executive committee is the restriction or termination of clinical privileges. This is understandably seen as a step attended by grave consequences for the practitioner in question with reference to his professional standing and to his ability to earn a living. The restriction of privileges is so serious that recommending it in response to a physician's habitual failure to justify all of the tests ordered for his Medicare patients may seem a little excessive. Yet his skimpy documentation or inefficient practice patterns will cost the hospital substantial amounts of money in the form of denied Medicare and other third-party payer claims. Unfortunately, however, the medical staff does not have at its disposal a convenient armamentarium of less damaging, more practical sanctions.

The content of most medical staff bylaws is related to a time when the only concerns that needed to be addressed in connection with the governance of the staff were related to professional ethics and competence. This has not changed materially for 50 years despite the fact that the economics of hospital care have changed dramatically. In 1930 a physician's tardiness in completing a medical record did not mean that the hospital would be unable to file a claim for reimbursement. Today medical staff members as a group are required to perform a variety of clerical and administrative tasks that were never contemplated in the design of traditional medical staff bylaws with their set of notably severe sanctions. For this reason, the principal sanctions that are available through the bylaws, designed as they were to deal with matters of ethical deviation and professional incompetence, are unsuitable for use in many situations today in which a physician's performance may violate hospital policy in ways that are independent of his ethical qualities and professional competence.

Given the anachronistic nature of medical staff bylaws and the extreme severity of the sanctions they provide, it is unrealistic to expect much in the way of performance analysis or modification through this apparatus. Responsibility for the assessment and analysis of patient care will have to be placed on the administrative structure of the hospital and its parent corporation.

The role of the medical staff in the quality assurance, risk control, and utilization control activities of the hospital should be an advisory one that is designed to enable the director of these programs to rely on the medical staff for guidance in clinical matters and for the formulation of clinical criteria for use in evaluation. The system that is currently in effect in many hospitals that place responsibility for hospital quality assurance in a medical staff committee cannot provide the strong direction required to ensure control of quality, utilization, and risk.

The Role of the Administrator

A major problem confronting the administrator vis-à-vis the issues of quality assurance, utilization control, and risk control is the lack of a clear definition of his authority in these areas. For example, the nursing service and ancillary services involved in patient care report to the administrator. Therefore, the administrator should be kept informed of the results of evaluation studies so he can take corrective action if needed. Yet in many hospitals quality monitoring reports involving nursing or ancillary personnel never reach an administrative officer who has the authority to make decisions on the basis of these studies. Quality assessment reports that contain even slightly unfavorable findings tend to be referred from one committee to another for months at a time.

In such hospital documents as the corporate bylaws and the medical staff bylaws, the accountability of the medical staff to the board of trustees is formally acknowledged. However, the typical organization chart of the community hospital depicts the administrator and the president or chief of the medical staff on the same level. The administrator is connected to the board by a solid line, while the medical staff president is rather vaguely affiliated with the administrator and the board by a series of dashed lines. This implies that the relationships are open to various interpretations, one being that these people sometimes talk to one another.

Under the existing relatively autonomous self-governing structure of the medical staff in most voluntary hospitals, the medical staff quality review committee usually feels no obligation to keep the administrator informed as to its findings from clinically-oriented evaluation studies. Exceptions to this policy occur in cases where the findings are so serious and have such potentially catastrophic implications that they may threaten the credibility and professional standing of any committee member who might try to ignore them or to deal with them covertly.

Recognizing their dependence on medical staff members to keep their hospitals occupied, administrators have usually backed off from the possibility of confrontation with respect to quality assurance issues, leaving the initiative to the medical staff, nursing service, and the heads of professional departments.

This lack of clarity as to the administrative responsibility for quality assurance is coupled with the fact that until two or three years ago few hospitals made explicit budgetary provisions for this activity. Such quality review work as was performed was not budgeted in terms of either labor-hours or funds. Nursing and ancillary service personnel were and still are expected to gather data, perform statistical analyses, and prepare reports during nonexistent spare time or during time taken away from their regularly scheduled duties. The services of outside consultants are often utilized for purposes of technical planning and training, but such services usually are supported by funds from an administrator's discretionary or contingency fund.

The budget plans of many—perhaps most—community hospitals do not provide for the quality assurance activity even though it has been a JCAH accreditation requirement since the early 1970s. In other words, hospitals are still trying to decide how to define the activity and where to position it in the organization. Since so many hospitals do not budget for patient care evaluation activities, they are not in a position to report any reliable expense figures for such activities. This situation casts serious doubt on the reliability of patient care evaluation expenses as they are reported to the Hospital Administrative Services program of the American Hospital Association.

This situation is quite different from the one found in other industries. The Ford Motor Company places responsibility for quality control on a divisional vice president of each division. These division vice presidents for quality control meet once each month with the corporation's president and quality control consultant. Responsibility for implementing quality control procedures is clearly defined throughout the organization. The quality control staff is directly accountable to the respective division vice presidents who have enough authority to relate directly to the operating vice presidents.

At International Harvester the program is called product reliability. The quality control staff of each product group reports to a vice president whose responsibilities include product reliability. Their findings provide the input for his recommendations to the operating vice presidents. Chrysler and General Motors follow a similar pattern of vesting responsibility for product reliability in the upper echelons of division or group management. All of these arrangements reflect corporate management's understanding of the tremendous financial importance of quality assurance.

Quality assurance is no less vital in the health care field. The overall responsibility for implementing the hospital governing body's policies with respect to quality of care must be vested in the hospital's or the system's chief executive officer. Where the chief executive officer of a community hospital is the administrator, the director of hospitalwide quality assurance, risk control, and utilization control programs should report directly to him. In a system that includes more than one facility, the local hospital's director of quality assurance should report directly to the corporate vice president who is responsible for quality assurance, risk control, and utilization control at the system level.

The Role of Professional Patient Care Personnel

In the typical hospital quality assurance program, nonphysician professional health care personnel are required to perform such tasks as data gathering, statistical analysis, and report preparation in addition to their regular duties. Further, in many instances they must carry out this survey work without receiving adequate training in the techniques involved.

From the practical standpoint, this lack of training and experience in evaluation research results in significant delays, technical difficulties, and added expense in implementing the quality assurance program. The hours of time diverted from direct patient care to perform these tasks that are required to meet the Joint Commission's quality assurance standards are not trivial in terms of payroll expense. Hospitals participating in the Hospital Administrative Services program of the American Hospital Association have reported patient care evaluation expenses averaging from $2.20 to $2.50 per discharge unit. However, the base used in these calculations is the direct expense that is attributable to an office and to a single quality assurance coordinator. For a more realistic estimate of the expense, it would be necessary to include the salary expense incurred in using such professional personnel as nurses and technologists to perform survey work.

The Joint Commission has always attempted to fill the training gap that exists in the hospital industry with respect to quality assessment. It conducts well-designed training programs for physicians and other hospital personnel in the techniques of departmental performance evaluation, but it is fighting an uphill battle. Until fairly recently, for example, a large part of the program content addressed to medical staff members had to consist of inspirational and motivational material. Before they could deal with the actual procedural material, the presenters had to convince the audience of the validity of the whole concept of objective performance evaluation as it applied to patient care.

While good training seminars and workshops in assessment techniques and procedures are available to nonphysician hospital personnel, the economics of the field are such that only a small percentage of those who must carry out the evaluation studies can participate in the training. Assuming that a community hospital with 150 beds has approximately 50 nonphysician health care personnel who are expected to participate in quality assurance activities, it is highly improbable that the hospital's budget would permit the administrator to send more than a dozen of them to survey-training workshops during the year. Furthermore, quality assurance workshops must compete for the continuing education dollar with a variety of other educational offerings, many of which are required for the members of the health care professions.

Maintaining an in-house training program is feasible under certain circumstances. Such a program, however, must function on an ongoing basis because of the relatively high turnover in some hospital occupations. It is most efficient and cost-effective in large hospitals where the services of a permanent educator can be justified. It is not cost-effective in small hospitals.

Since, in most hospitals, it is not realistic or cost-effective to train hospital personnel in survey design and implementation, the most practical solution is to establish an office of quality assurance, risk control, and utilization control as described earlier and to staff it with one or more full-time employees who report to the director of the combined programs. In the model program described in the next few chapters, this organizational unit is referred to as the office of standards. Its head is referred to as the director of standards.

As in the case of the medical staff, the heads of nursing service and ancillary departments or units should participate in the program in an advisory capacity. They should be responsible for developing relevant criteria for use in the evaluation studies of their respective departments or services. Data collection, data analysis, and report preparation should be performed by the employees of the office of standards. Employing clinical staff in such tasks is neither productive nor cost-effective.

4

The Quality Assurance Program: Objectives, Structure, and Scope

The Joint Commission increasingly emphasizes the need for placing responsibility for quality assurance activity in a centralized agency within the hospital. The most recent revision of the quality assurance standard also emphasizes continuous monitoring of patient care where emphasis was formerly on problem-focused retrospective review.

In this and the next several chapters, a representative model plan for performing quality review and management will be outlined. Such a plan can be broken down into the following segments:

Objectives.

Structure.

Scope and coverage.

Implementation and evaluation research methodology.

Impact of evaluation studies.

Evaluation of the effects.

45

The Objectives

The principal objectives of the combined program in quality assurance, risk control, and utilization control are

- Maintenance of high levels of quality in patient care within the fiscal constraints imposed by the prospective payment system.
- Protection of the hospital's reimbursement claims.
- Containment of hospital costs.
- Protection of the hospital's financial assets.

It might be appropriate to add another objective to the list that reflects the competitive needs of the hospital in a recently tight, competitive market. This would be product differentiation. In light of new competition not only from other hospitals but also from physicians' offices and a variety of ambulatory care facilities, it would be to the hospital's advantage to demonstrate in some way that its standards of care are superior.

In the area of risk control, quality assurance serves to minimize exposure to risks of malpractice thereby protecting the hospital's assets and preventing experience-related increases in malpractice insurance premiums.

Obviously, the considerations of good medical practice inherently dictate the minimization of complications in patients. However, there is now an additional financial consideration that has an impact on hospital operating margins. Under the prospective payment plan the hospital may have to absorb the expenses resulting from an extended stay due to complications in the treatment of federally funded patients. Therefore, hospitals must strive to identify and eliminate the causes of hospital-related complications of care. Quality assurance in the service of preventing complications functions to contain the costs of hospital care.

The following is an example of a statement of purpose that is suitable for inclusion in the written quality assurance plan.

Objectives and Means

The objective of the Quality Assurance Plan of _____ Hospital is the preservation and enhancement of the high quality of patient care in part by ensuring that

1. Patient care personnel are qualified and effectively supervised.

2. Patient care services are appropriately organized with clear channels of supervision, responsibility, and accountability.

3. Care that is appropriate to the needs of patients is delivered in a timely manner, is optimal within the range of available resources, is consistent with achievable goals, and is properly documented.

4. Patient care is delivered in as cost-effective a manner as is possible.

5. Documentation facilitates the continuity of care and the evaluation of services.

6. All elements entering into the care of patients are subjected to periodic review, retrospective or concurrent, with the use of preestablished objective criteria and documentation of the findings.

7. The findings of patient care review are utilized by the hospital in concrete ways to fulfill the objectives of the Quality Assurance Program.

It is the responsibility of the Board of Trustees to establish, maintain, and support, through the Chief Executive Officer and the Chairman of the Medical Staff, an ongoing Quality Assurance Program that includes effective mechanisms for reviewing and evaluating patient care and that provides for effective responses to the findings of such an evaluation. Toward this end the Hospital has established the Quality Assurance Function as a standing or continuous monitoring and corrective action program of the administration and professional staffs. The following activities are incorporated in the Quality Assurance Program:

1. Identification of potential problems or concerns in the delivery of health care services.

2. Objective assessment of the cause and scope of each problem.

3. Implementation of decisions and plans designed to resolve observed problems.

4. Monitoring of activities designed to ensure that the desired results have been achieved.

5. Documentation substantiating the effectiveness of the program in improving patient care and ensuring sound clinical performance.

6. Reporting of findings to the Medical Staff, the Chief Executive Officer, and the Board of Trustees.

7. Annual appraisal of the effectiveness of the Quality Assurance Program.

The means to be employed for the purpose of achieving these objectives set forth above will encompass evaluation research and corrective action, as is described in later sections of this document.

The Structure of the Program

This is the most vital aspect of the entire program. Once the goals of the quality assurance program have been established, it is necessary to set up an organization structure that will be adequate for mobilizing and channeling the efforts of the people who are to be held accountable for the results of the enterprise. The authors of the plan must clearly identify by title those individuals who are responsible for directing, supervising, reviewing, or performing the specific tasks that are to be assigned in later sections of the written quality assurance plan. The authors should avoid using generalities such as "members of the medical staff" or "the administration." Responsibility must be clearly assigned if the apparatus is to work.

Supervisory responsibilities and accountability must be set forth with precision. Each person involved in a quality assurance activity must know to whom he or she reports on quality assurance matters as well as the nature and extent of his or her own supervisory authority. These matters can be dealt with in summary fashion in the plan, and each participant should receive a brief memorandum from the director of the office of standards providing more specifics as to his or her own duties.

Sample provisions from a model plan that contemplates the existence of a single office of quality assurance, risk control, and utilization control follow.

Structure of the Quality Assurance Program

General direction of the quality assurance program shall be the responsibility of the Board of Trustees' Committee on Quality Assurance, Risk Control, and Utilization Control.

The Medical Staff, through its Credentials Committee, shall be responsible for reviewing and evaluating all applications for membership and renewal of membership on the Medical Staff; for making recommendations to the Board of Trustees concerning appointment and reappointment to the Medical Staff; and for making recommendations to the Board of Trustees concerning the delineation, expansion, restriction, or suspension of clinical privileges.

The Medical Staff will strive to ensure, through its ongoing monitoring and review of patient care, that the highest level of quality in such care is maintained. The quality review and assurance activities provided for in the Medical Staff Bylaws are hereby incorporated by reference in the Quality Assurance Plan.

The Chief Executive Officer of the Hospital is accountable to the Board of Trustees for the effective organizational and operational development of the quality assurance program and for ensuring successful implementation of the quality assurance plan. The Chief Executive Officer shall be responsible for keeping the Committee on Standards fully informed, by means of reports at Committee meetings, on review and monitoring findings relating to all aspects of the quality of patient care in the Hospital.

Together with the Executive Committee of the Medical Staff, or their designees, the Chief Executive Officer and the Director of Standards shall develop guidelines for the purpose of defining incentive measures, sanctions, and appropriate corrective action for the resolution of performance problems that have an impact on the quality of patient care in the hospital.

Full administrative responsibility for the quality assurance program of the Hospital is vested in the Director of Standards, who shall report to the Hospital's Chief Executive Officer.

The Office of Standards shall be staffed with professional and clerical personnel in numbers sufficient to perform the duties of the Office. If Quality Assurance or Utilization Review Coordinators are employed by the Hospital, they will be a part of the staff of this Office, and will report to the Director of Standards.

With respect to administering the quality assurance program, the principal responsibilities and duties of the Director shall include, but shall not be limited to, the following:

1. To ensure that by December 1 of each year the President of the Medical Staff and the head of each clinical and administrative department or service in the Hospital has appointed a representative to serve during the coming calendar year as that unit's liaison with the Office in connection with such activities as the collection of data and the development of evaluation criteria for monitoring patient care.
2. To establish and maintain an annual schedule of monitoring projects together with a reporting schedule.
    To maintain the schedule establishing target dates for the submission of topics and criteria by the Medical Staff, departments, and services.
3. Following consultation with the respective appointed Medical Staff, department, and service representatives, to design evaluation research

projects that will be conducted in accordance with the schedule.

a. To develop hypotheses to guide the research process.

b. To identify the types of data to be collected.

c. To identify appropriate sources of needed data.

d. To identify the appropriate statistical methods to be employed in the analysis.

e. To design the statistical and graphic displays that will be appropriate to the study.

f. To assign the tasks of data collection, analysis, and report preparation to staff of the Office.

g. To review all staff activities in data collection, statistical analysis, and report preparation.

h. To review the findings of each project with the head and liaison representative of the department or service involved.

i. To develop recommendations for corrective action as needed.

4. To submit to the Chief Executive Officer executive reports, including recommendations, on all monitoring activities.

5. To plan and schedule follow-up studies to determine the impact of the recommendations for corrective action.

6. In the absence of problem resolution, to refer the problem to the Chief Executive Officer along with an executive summary, supporting documentation, and recommendations.

The President of the Medical Staff, the Director of Nursing Services, and the head of each administrative and clinical department or service in the Hospital's organization shall appoint, by December 1 of each year, a member of the staff, department, or service to serve during the coming calendar year as a representative to and liaison with the Office of Standards. The principal responsibilities of the representatives in implementing the quality assurance plan will be the identification of problem areas in patient care and other subjects for evaluation monitoring as well as the development of objective, measurable criteria for use in such monitoring activities.

Note that the section on program structure in the model provisions above contains no reference to the quality assurance committee of the medical staff. The reason is that this committee's establishment is a matter for medical staff determination, whereas the quality assurance plan developed here is addressed essentially to corporate responsibilities. The medical staff's quality assurance or patient care review committee would be provided for in the medical staff bylaws rather than in a corporate document such as the hospital's quality assurance plan. The role of the medical staff quality review committee would be advisory. Presumably, the medical staff representation provided for in the quality assurance plan would be one of the activities of the medical staff's quality assurance or patient care review committee.

The Scope of the Program

Activities to Be Covered

Quality review should be broad in its coverage, including patients representing the major diagnostic categories seen in the hospital. The written quality assurance plan should provide for the assessment of both inpatient and outpatient services.

In addition it is to the hospital's advantage to include administrative services in its quality assessment program. Satisfactory levels of productivity are measures of good quality of performance. This aspect of the organization's overall operation should be considered. The same approaches apply in the measurement of both quality of care and productivity.

A suitable quality assurance plan provision might include the following language:

Services Covered

All services that influence the care of patients will be included in the Quality Assurance Program. Such services and groups include, but are not limited to, the following:

1. Administration.
2. Ambulatory care, including clinics and outpatient services.
3. Anesthesia services.
4. Central services.
5. Clinical laboratories.
6. Emergency services or department.
7. Environmental services, including maintenance, engineering, housekeeping, and laundry.
8. Food services.
9. Medical records services.
10. Medical staff.
11. Nuclear medicine services.
12. Nursing services.
13. Pathology services.
14. Pharmacy services.
15. Physical therapy services.
16. Prenatal clinic.
17. Radiology services.
18. Respiratory therapy services.
19. Safety and risk management services.
20. Social services.

Types of Review to Be Performed

In determining the types of review to be performed, three issues should be considered: (1) time frames, (2) subject matter, and (3) data sources to be utilized.

Time Frames. The choice of a time frame depends largely on the nature of the data to be collected. In a study addressed chiefly to the presence or absence of specified indications for admission or for admission to a particular type of unit, prospective screening may be appropriate.

If the medical staff and hospital policy emphasize the use of preadmission diagnostic workups for patients scheduled for elective surgery, prospective screening on this criterion is appropriate and very useful.

Where the subject under investigation is the performance of certain specified procedures for a given class of patients in accordance with a prescribed schedule, it would be most useful to conduct concurrent monitoring, probably at the nursing stations or zones, or at the sites at which the procedures are normally performed. Generic screening with concurrent data gathering is also a useful approach. Certainly, where the collection of data must be done by direct observation—as in evaluating technical performance—the monitoring must be concurrent.

Concurrent monitoring through observation is often the only practical approach to data gathering in studies dealing with, for example, housekeeping practices, infection control techniques, or the insertion of intravenous needles or of catheters.

In tracing behavior that is assumed to be associated with some definable outcome that has been identified in a sample of patients, a retrospective review involving the collection of data from medical records and other documents may be most useful. A properly documented retrospective review cannot be performed, of course, where recorded data are not available for retrieval.

Subject Matter. Valuable time and effort should not be wasted on studies of trivial problems that could be readily resolved through timely administrative action. In other words, thorough assessment surveys should be reserved for those problems that are associated with genuine disagreement or uncertainty as to causation and accompanied by potentially serious consequences for patients, staff, or visitors. Performing a review study is no substitute for appropriate administrative decision making. Rather, its purpose is to provide the information needed to illuminate decision making.

Subjects on which it is appropriate to conduct evaluation reviews have the following characteristics:

1. They relate to behavior that has a significant effect on the welfare of patients, staff, or visitors.
2. They reflect behavior that either has been recorded or on

which it is possible to collect data concurrently or prospectively.

3. The consequences of continued deviation from hospital policy or criteria include the suboptimal care of patients, financial loss on denied claims, jeopardy to the hospital's accreditation, jeopardy to the hospital's licensure and health department approvals, and the hazards of exposure to malpractice or personal injury claims.

4. It is necessary to document causal relationships in order to facilitate decision making with respect to the development of procedural guidelines.

These four points include no reference to the fact that it should be possible to develop criteria for evaluation of the activity under review. This omission is deliberate. While objective criteria for the assessment of many activities may not be found in the medical and nursing literature, it has been the author's experience that, in the health care field, knowledgeable individuals can always formulate and verbalize the criteria they apply in making judgments as to the appropriateness or relative value of various procedures and results. The process of articulating implicit criteria may take a little time, but the exercise is practical and worthwhile.

Data Sources to Be Utilized

Incident reports that are generated through the risk control system are increasingly being used as indicators of possible problems that demand study. This is a healthy trend—one that can be expected to contribute to the value of quality review. Utilization review documents can be used to point out unjustified admissions, inappropriate resource application, and complication-generated extended hospital stays.

Other useful sources of data include not only medical records and other documents but the hospital environment itself. Although they are data collection methods rather than data sources, observation and interview must not be overlooked when a study is being planned.

The following provisions are taken from a model quality assurance plan that reflects common current policies:

Types of Review

The Quality Assurance Program is implemented through the performance of a variety of analytical studies of the nature and quality of patient care services and the manner in which they are delivered. While patient care evaluation studies may be either retrospective or concurrent, it is advisable, where possible, to employ concurrent monitoring in data collection. Generic screening with concurrent data gathering is one method that will be used as indicated. Where problems in patient care or in the delivery of care have been identified, they should be addressed in the monitoring process.

The principal sources of data used in this process will include, but need not be limited to, current and completed medical records, departmental records, utilization review records, activity profiles, incident reports, treatment records, hospital billing records, and the records of the preventive maintenance and safety inspections of plant and equipment.

A study may be addressed to the problems that arise in connection with a diagnosis, a procedure, a treatment modality, or the operation of a department or service. Identification of suitable topics may be based on evidence of problems that were revealed in previous studies and JCAH surveys as well as on the observations and insights of members of the various professional staffs and services.

Review criteria will be based on such entities as national and regional norms, statistical norms developed on the basis of the Hospital's own experience, and consensual definitions of optimal or ideal performance.

5

Evaluation Research in the Program: Definition and Hypothesis

Implementation of a quality assurance plan entails two basic activities: evaluation research and corrective action. Evaluation research is the process of defining and investigating some segment of activity that is to be measured against preestablished criteria. If, as a result of the research, significant variations from the criteria are found, the organization may take the next step—instituting some set of measures designed to correct the variations.

Evaluation Research

The process of evaluation research formally involves the following steps:

- Defining the activity to be studied.
- Developing a hypothesis to guide the investigation.
- Defining the study sample.
- Identifying the data sources.
- Developing criteria against which to compare the retrieved data.

- Collecting and analyzing the data.
- Preparing a report that includes the conclusions from the analysis.
- Designing and performing a follow-up study.

Since taking corrective action is not a part of evaluation research, discussion of that issue is deferred for the present.

The Process of Defining the Activity to Be Studied

Delivery of Services

The fragmentation of review activities in hospitals makes it difficult for personnel to identify or define those aspects of patient care that must be reviewed or monitored. The surface effects seen at the unit level often obscure an underlying problem. Each department, service, or committee sees a restricted aspect of patient services by studying a limited sample of events in which it has taken part and retrieving data only from its own records. This investigation approach has been described before—in fables about people examining elephants and in common observations about the true size of icebergs. It is an inevitable result of encouraging each of the many organizational units in a hospital to conduct its own studies without reference to those planned or performed by other groups. A major, common problem is the failure to utilize data from as many sources as possible.

Examples of this are numerous. The executive director of a large midwestern medical center requested assistance in resolving what he perceived to be an operating problem due to an excessive number of transfers. The matter was brought to his attention by the director of management information services. She was unable to arrive at what she considered to be a reliable midnight census figure due to discrepancies in admission and discharge data that were forwarded to her office every 24 hours. The problem was believed to be in the admitting office's documentation practices.

An on-site preliminary investigation elicited some additional findings.

- Attending physicians frequently complained that as a result of in-house patient transfers, they wasted a great deal of time trying to find their patients while making rounds each day.

- The pharmacy and laboratories wasted many hours (eventually, this was fully documented) of employee time each week trying to locate patients in order to deliver medications, obtain specimens, and return laboratory reports.

- The dietetic service complained about the large numbers of trays that were returned each day, because the patients for whom they were intended could not be found. At the same time, the service was kept busy supplying replacement trays for patients whose trays had been delivered to the wrong rooms. In addition, on the day and evening shifts, trays were provided, in an alcove off the main lobby, for patients who were waiting to be admitted to rooms that were still occupied, even though discharge records indicated that they were empty. While the actual annual costs of the misdirected and replaced trays were not a large portion of this institution's annual budget, the situation was interfering with the efficient operation of the dietetic department and was a symptom of a more serious problem.

- Delays in receiving laboratory and radiology reports at nursing zones often resulted in an extra day's preoperative stay for a patient or in an extra day's stay beyond the day on which he was to be discharged. Claims for the extra days to the Medicare fiscal intermediary and other third-party payers were being denied. The result was that the hospital had to absorb the unreimbursed expenses or try to recoup them from the patients.

- The number of rooms that had to be prepared for new admissions or transfers after 5:30 P.M. was so great that the director of housekeeping services had to maintain a full crew of roommakers on the second shift.

An analysis of all of these separately reported events pointed to one underlying factor, the effect of which was exacerbated by two or three other behavioral patterns that characterized the hospital's operations. The fundamental problem was the fact that although the medical center did have a liberal, written and published discharge policy of long standing, specifying that patients were to leave their rooms by 11:00 A.M. on the day of discharge, the policy had never been observed.

Among the reasons cited by hospital personnel for failure to enforce this policy was the fact that many of their patients came in from rural areas, which, although not exactly remote, are as much as an hour's drive from the hospital. Therefore, their relatives did not find it convenient to call for them until after the completion of the day's work on the farm or at their place of business. This accounts for the fact that many of these patients did not actually leave the premises until seven or eight hours after they had been officially discharged. Nursing service personnel, who were sympathetic to an elderly, frail patient, often did not wish to send such an individual downstairs to wait alone in the lobby. Thus the patient was encouraged to remain in the room. However, there was also a temptation to hoard patients until after the end of the first shift.

Another contributing factor was that many of the medical staff members did not understand that insurance coverage did not extend beyond the stated checkout time on the day of discharge as this was recorded in the medical record. In other words, although they wrote their discharge orders on, for example, January 15, scheduling discharge for the following day, they often told the patient that the room was "paid for" until midnight of the following day—there was no reason to hurry the departure. The patient accounts office reported the prevalence of this misunderstanding.

Another common reason for delays in discharge was the fact that the attending physician often did not wish to write the discharge order until he had an opportunity to review the final laboratory or radiology reports. If these reports were 24 hours late in reaching the patient's zone, because the patient had to be traced and located, that meant an additional day's stay.

Finally, additional observation and interviews revealed that the nurses about to go off duty at 3:00 P.M. simply did not wish to become involved in all of the administrative tasks involved in receiving new admissions between, say, 2:00 and 3:00 P.M. Therefore, they hoarded those patients who were still on the floors thus hiding from the housekeeping service and the admitting office the fact that they had been discharged. This had the effect of stacking up patients waiting to be admitted, many of whom waited for five or more hours. The consequences of this practice for the housekeeping and dietetic departments have already been described. The nursing shift coming on duty at 3:00 P.M. then faced the task of admitting the backlog of patients and ordering their dinner and breakfast trays.

These findings explained why rooms were often unavailable for patients who were waiting to be admitted. This still did not explain why so many patient transfers were taking place.

The hospital had a clearly stated policy on admission times. Elective and urgent admissions were supposed to take place before 2:00 P.M. This policy had been ignored for as long as anyone could remember. Patients routinely arrived for elective admissions at any time of the day, with many arriving as late as 5:30 P.M. In fact, admitting office personnel stated that many patients arrived at the center without any previous notice from their physicians. Local physicians were in the habit of advising their patients to "Go over to the hospital and tell them that I want you admitted."

The reason for the failure to comply? Back in the 1950s, when the first building of the center was erected, its administration feared competition from another good hospital in the same town. The two facilities shared essentially the same medical staff. As a marketing tactic, the administration of the medical center readily made many concessions to the medical staff. One of these concessions was the willingness to admit patients at any time.

The nursing service was responsible for assigning patients to units and rooms. When a patient arrived for admission, the admitting office staff contacted the nursing service to obtain an appropriate room assignment. This was done because the hospital maintained a strict system of patient categorization by diagnostic group and level of care required. However, when the admitting physician did not alert the admitting office as to the arrival of the patient, the whole admission and categorization process had to be suspended while hospital personnel located the physician to determine the patient's diagnosis and the level of care required.

In addition to this categorization, two other assignment systems were in operation. One reflected the desire of the attending physicians to have their patients grouped together in contiguous areas of the hospital. This facilitated making rounds. The desire was understandable, because the six-story building occupies an entire square block of ground space. However, since a number of the medical staff members were family practitioners and general practitioners, they may have been seeing patients with a variety of diagnoses at any given time.

The other assignment system provided for placement due to nonmedical reasons that were not related to the physician clustering policy. The large main building includes a new wing that was built in about 1979. This wing is considered by local people to be more desirable than the older part of the hospital, although there are no differences in the room rates. The decor and amenities vary only slightly. The 30-year-old portion of the building has been very well maintained. The hospital contains no shared rooms in either the old section or the new wing. Nonetheless, it was found that many patients who were assigned to rooms in the older section asked upon admission to be transferred to the first available room in the new section—and the nursing service tried to accommodate their wishes.

Thus with admissions occurring throughout the first shift and in the first half of the second shift and discharged patients continuing to occupy rooms—often until midafternoon—the nursing service routinely found it necessary to "bump" patients in order to assign incoming patients to rooms according to the categorization system.

As a result of lax admission and discharge policies combined with attempts to adhere to a patient categorization system while bowing to requests for nonmedically indicated transfers, patients were continually being transferred. Inspection of admitting office records disclosed countless instances of patients who were transferred twice in 24 hours, excluding patients who were transferred in or out of special care units or the surgical section.

This account is offered as an example of a problem in the delivery of patient services that generated data relating to many different services of the hospital. Information reflecting the impact of the problem was supplied by the medical staff, the nursing service, the housekeeping department, the dietetic service, the pharmacy, the laboratories, the radiology service, the admitting office, the management information and data processing services, and the medical record department. Resolving the problem became a joint project on the parts of the medical staff, the nursing service, and the admitting office.

Where quality research is carried on by a single unit in the organization, it is possible to monitor and synthesize information from all of the clinical and administrative divisions, observing trends and shared patterns. This is far more efficient than the fragmented approach.

Medical Care and Medical Staff Review Activity

In addition to requiring as a condition of accreditation that hospitals maintain formal quality assurance programs covering all patient care–related activities and performance, the Joint Commission on Accreditation of Hospitals requires that the hospital's organized medical staff monitor its own performance in certain specified areas. In other words, this review is to be performed as a study of each of the specified activity areas, whether or not any problems can be identified.

In order to comply with JCAH standards, the hospital must be able to document that this self-monitoring activity is maintained by the medical staff in accordance with a schedule established in the medical staff chapter of the Accreditation Manual for Hospitals.

The following provision in the hospital's quality assurance plan reflects the 1984 JCAH standards requirement:

Medical Staff Review

The office of standards performs the following specified studies for review by the medical staff in accordance with the schedules that follow. All monitoring and evaluation studies entail the use of preestablished written criteria formulated by representatives of the services covered.

Monitoring and Evaluation of the Quality and Appropriateness of Patient Care Provided by All Individuals with Clinical Privileges. Monitoring and evaluation involving the routine collection of data on important aspects of patient care are performed and reported on a monthly basis. The reports with findings are referred to the medical staff for the development of recommendations designed to bring about the solution of any problems observed.

Through its designated representative, the medical staff provides a monthly report on any problem-solving actions taken.

Antibiotic Utilization Review. Reports on the utilization of antibiotics are prepared for the medical staff on at least a quarterly basis.

Blood Utilization Review. Reports on the use of blood and blood products are prepared for the medical staff on at least a quarterly basis.

Medical Record Review. While the medical records of many patients are reviewed in the course of the monitoring of patient care, the records are analyzed and evaluated as documents per se on a quarterly basis. In the course of this review, the structure, format, and content of the records are evaluated with reference to their use in the hospital's data base as well as to the quality of the data. Reports on this review are submitted to the medical staff on a quarterly basis.

Pharmacy and Therapeutics Review. Reports on pharmacy and therapeutics reviews, including studies concerning the indications for and utilization of any new drugs being introduced, are prepared for the medical staff on a quarterly basis.

Surgical Case Review. Surgical case review is conducted on a monthly basis and reported to the medical staff. The review includes cases in which no specimens were submitted to the pathologist.

While the language of the Joint Commission's 1984 standards interpretations suggests that the specified reviews are intended as evaluation studies, personnel in many hospitals apparently do not interpret the standard in this way. For example, in many hospitals the medical staff review of the utilization of antibiotics consists merely of a tabulation of the numbers of cultures that were obtained, the numbers of doses of specified antibiotics that were administered during the month, and a report on the presence or absence of reactions. It is unusual to find any comparison in these reports with preestablished criteria for indications. In many such reports there is no evidence that the investigator even sought to determine whether the antibiotics given were consistent with the culture and sensitivity findings.

The report on the utilization of blood and blood products in many hospitals consists of a listing of the number of units administered, the number of single unit transfusions, and the presence or absence of reactions. In many hospitals the blood utilization reports contain no reference to the presence or absence of indications for transfusions or for the particular blood component utilized.

If the required medical staff review studies were performed by a central office responsible for all evaluation research in the hospital, these flaws in the studies could be eliminated. The specific medical staff review studies would be designed to follow the same format as similar studies of other services and activities. They would employ preestablished written evaluation criteria. In addition the studies would be designed to focus on potential or established problems.

The Hypothesis

Before constructing the study sample, identifying data sources, and formulating review criteria, it is advisable to devise a simple hypothesis to provide a possible explanation of the problem to be studied. Having to state assumptions and to project causal relationships forces the investigator to organize his thoughts on the subject. With a hypothesis to test, he is in a better position to decide on the size and composition of the sample, the most productive sources of data, and the criteria against which the observed performance is to be compared. The hypothesis provides a frame of reference, and setting it up before designing the study usually saves a lot of time by preventing errors and the need for repetition of work.

The hypothesis should be neither elaborate nor complex. If it's complex the investigator will probably have more than one study to perform. The following is an example of one type of simple, testable hypothesis:

The Problem. It was found, in the course of a retrospective study on another subject, that in many cases in which antibiotics were administered, the drugs were changed within a day or two of the initial order. None of the medical records involved contained explicit reports or descriptions of drug reactions. Some patients received more than two different antibiotics in succession. None of the physicians treating these patients was in the habit of ordering sensitivity tests along with the orders for cultures.

Possible Causes

1. The attending physicians did not know that it was necessary in that hospital to write an order specifically for sensitivity testing.
2. The attending physicians considered the added expense of the sensitivity test to be unwarranted.
3. The antibiotics that were initially ordered were inappropriate for use in the infections that were present and were ineffective as treatment.
4. Drug reactions had occurred but had not been described as such in the progress notes or nursing notes.

Hypothesis to Be Tested. In the absence of sensitivity reports, the drugs that were initially ordered were ineffective against the organisms cultured.

Although one hypothesis was formulated to guide the criterion development and identification of data sources, it would be appropriate to collect any data available in the records dealing with possible cause number 4 as well.

6

Evaluation Research in the Program: Sampling and Data Sources

In this chapter the discussion will center on the next tasks in an evaluation research project: constructing the study sample and identifying sources of data for use in monitoring. These items were identified in the evaluation research process in Chapter 5.

The Sample: Probability Sampling

The balance of this discussion relates to the construction of probability sampling plans. The explanations are designed to assist the individual who is responsible for planning the sampling in a quality assurance program. Characteristics of probability sampling plans include the following:

- Every member of the population from which the sample is drawn has a known probability of being included. Note that this is not the same as saying that every member has the same probability of being included.

- The sample is drawn by some method of random selection that is consistent with these known probabilities.

- In making estimates on the basis of the sample, the investigator takes into account the known probabilities of selection.

The first thing about which most investigators in hospital quality assurance concern themselves is the size of the sample to be used in a study. There is no magic size for a sample. A 10 percent sample is not necessarily twice as good as a 5 percent sample. It depends on several factors that should enter into the decision about sample size and composition.

Two primary considerations to be addressed when planning the data collection are

1. How big a sample can you afford to use? Labor costs are generated in data collection, and your office of standards operates within a budget. Its payroll expenses must be allocated over the entire array of studies that it performs each year.

2. At what level of confidence do you wish to be able to make assertions or predictions about the class of events or groups of patients under study? For most purposes in the social sciences, a confidence level of 95 percent is considered acceptable. This means that your estimate of the mean value of some attribute or characteristic of the population sampled will be correct—except for what you define as the "allowable error"—95 out of 100 times.

In order to be able to use either of the common formulas for determining the needed sample size, you need to have two values. One value is known as the allowable error. This value is simply the size of error in the estimate that the users of the study results are willing to accept, with the understanding that 95 out of 100 times the size of the error will be no greater than that specified. The allowable error is expressed as a range of values above and below the estimated mean. Since it relates to the peculiarities of the events being studied, the allowable error should be determined by personnel who are involved in the type of hospital service being reviewed.

The other numerical value that is needed to determine sample size under certain conditions is an estimate of the population standard deviation. This is a measure of the dispersion of the values of an attribute about its mean value in the population from which you will draw a sample. This parameter is needed in constructing samples for the study of variables that are assumed to follow the pattern known as the normal distribution, which is shown graphically as the familiar bell-shaped curve. An example of the calculation using an estimate of the population standard deviation is shown below.

Let n = sample size,
 σ = the population standard deviation,
 L = the allowable error,
       and the desired confidence limit is 95%.

$$n = \frac{4\sigma^2}{L^2}$$

It is difficult to use this method of determining sample size in studying hospital personnel behavior, because there is usually no available information on the size of the population standard deviation. If you are studying the occurrence of a clinical phenomenon, the medical or nursing literature may contain research reports giving the parameters of the distributions in other populations studied.

However, in most hospital quality assurance studies you will be working with events that can be described in terms of the binomial distribution; that is, they are either present or absent in the sample. This type of sample is used in the next example.

Assume that you have been asked by one of the hospital services to study the occurrence of a specific, defined procedural flaw in the performance of one of the treatments for which they are responsible. For study purposes you can consider the presence of this procedural flaw as an "event." The service's personnel have formulated two or three criteria against which you will compare data from a departmental log and medical records. You are to estimate the number of times this problem occurs so that they can decide what kind of corrective action is needed.

Assume that the service has decided that the allowable error in estimating the occurrence of this event is 10 percent. In other words, they won't object if your estimate deviates as much as 10 percent from the true figure, provided that there is only a 5 percent chance of its being more than 10 percent off. Incidentally, the procedure under review was performed 8,000 times last year.

You feel that a study sample of 20 cases might very well miss some of those that should be reviewed. However, you don't have the budget to collect data on a 5 percent sample, or 400 cases. A simple formula will help to determine an appropriate sample size. This is a crude method of making this determination, but it is adequate in the absence of good data on the amount of variance in the overall population.

This approach depends on the fact that the occurrences in question follow a binomial distribution; that is, for your purposes, they are either present or absent from the data base. Therefore, you can use a calculation based on the chances of the occurrence of the procedural error being studied. Members of the service tell you that the chance of the error occurring in any given stack of records, or in any given record, are about even, or 50-50. For your calculation, then, this probability is expressed as "pq" = (50) (50).

Let n = sample size,
p = chance of error's being present = 50%,
q = chance of error's being absent = 50%,
and L = allowable error = 10%.

$$n = \frac{4(pq)}{L^2}$$

$n = 100$ cases.

The chance of an event occurring is not always 50 percent. The personnel of the service requesting the study might have told you that, on the basis of their experience, they would expect the procedural error to be found 20 percent of the time. In that case, the chances would be 20-80, and the sample size could be smaller.

In planning the sample to be used in a review study, it is important first to define the population about which you are going to make inferences or projections and from which the sample will be drawn. For example, do you want to learn something about the care given to all male patients over the age of 65 or about the care given to male patients over 65 who were being treated for pneumonia? Is your concern with the care of male patients over 65 who were treated for pneumonia between January 1 and

March 15? Is your interest in the care given to male patients over 65 who were treated for pneumonia with a particular type of antibiotic between January 1 and March 15?

For this discussion it will be assumed that you plan to use some form of probability sampling most of the time. There is one exception to this general practice. This exception occurs when the definition of the group about which information is sought is so refined, so narrow, that it turns out that the entire number of such patients or events was fewer than 30 during the previous 12 months. Where this is the case, it is practical to include the entire population in the study. For example, in a small midwestern hospital the pediatric service wished to conduct a retrospective review of the care of newborns with hyperbilirubinemia—a blood abnormality that sometimes occurs in newborns. When it was found that only 15 infants during the preceding 12 months had had this condition, the entire group of 15 was included in the study.

Except when you're dealing with a population that includes fewer than 20 individuals or events, the sample should not ordinarily be smaller than 20. When the estimated population is in the hundreds within the given time frame for the study, then it should be remembered that the calculation of the level of confidence to be associated with any estimates of means derived from the data involves the ratio of the standard error of the sample mean to the square root of the sample size. Therefore, the larger the sample and its square root, the lower this ratio and the higher the level of confidence with which you can make assertions about the study findings.

The sample size depends on the amount of variation of the values of the variable being studied around its mean value in the population and on the level of confidence that you wish to attach to your estimates. In addition you cannot ignore your data collection budget. The size of the population itself is not the controlling factor in choosing sample size. Variation within the population is far more important.

Bear in mind that the population referred to may be not only patients but such things as trays prepared by the dietetic service or orders processed by the pharmacy.

Three types of probability sampling are commonly used in studies of hospital care. These are:

Simple random sampling.

Systematic sampling.

Stratified random sampling.

Simple Random Sampling

Simple random sampling is useful and easy to carry out. You need a copy of a table of random numbers to start. Such tables are commonly found in college statistics textbooks. Assume that you have decided to use a sample of 20 patients and that your population consists of 200 patients discharged within some stated recent period. All patients, in order to be included in the population, share whatever attributes you have chosen to define the population. They can be numbered from 1 to 200 on the basis of their discharge dates.

In random number tables, the figures are arranged in columns of 5-digit numbers. Since your population is identified by a 3-digit number (200), you will be looking only at the last three digits of the 5-digit cluster you start with. Enter one of the columns on the page in any row you wish. Then, looking at the third, fourth, and fifth digits of each set of 5-digit numbers as you read down the column, select the first 20 3-digit numbers that do not exceed 200. Match these 20 numbers with the previously identified cases, which you have listed as Cases 1 to 200—that is your sample.

Systematic Sampling

In drawing a systematic sample, the first case number alone is chosen with the help of the table of random numbers. You simply choose the rest of the cases on the basis of a previously decided proportion of the population. Thus if you wish to draw 10 percent of the population for the sample, you will select every 10th case.

This method has two advantages over simple random sampling. It is easier with a large sample, because you do not need to refer to the table of random numbers after the first selection. In addition it tends to spread the sample more evenly over the entire population.

However, systematic sampling also has two significant disadvantages. First, when the population being studied exhibits some periodic or cyclic variation, and your selection cycle happens to coincide with that pattern, the pattern may occur in the sample, distorting the findings and leading to unwarranted conclusions. Second, if you are studying some variable for which you need to obtain a measurement, such as the mean value over the sample, there is no way to determine the standard error of the mean in a systematic sample. Therefore, you cannot determine the level of confidence with which the results can be reported.

You can deal with the first problem by carefully studying the characteristics of the original population before designing the sample. In this way, any periodicity can be detected and the selection pattern can be planned in such a way as to avoid the coincidence.

Stratified Sampling

Stratified sampling can be very useful in a hospital quality assurance application when certain conditions apply to the population. These are:

- The presence in the population of some defining characteristic, other than the attribute under investigation, that effectively serves to distinguish, in some significant way, some groups of the population members from other groups. Where you are dealing with a fairly large, heterogeneous sample, precision is gained by breaking the sample down into more nearly homogeneous subsamples, or strata.

- The fact that the variable being studied shows a highly skewed distribution, making it unrealistic, for example, to rely on a value such as the mean for the entire population. One professor of population statistics used to illustrate this hazard with the story of the statistician who drowned in a river with an average depth of 12 inches.

Other advantages, such as overcoming data collecting difficulties in different subgroups in the sample (strata), usually do not apply in hospital settings.

In constructing a stratified sample, the entire heterogeneous sample is divided into homogeneous groups called strata, and a sample is drawn independently and randomly from each stratum. The strata need not be the same size. In fact, this is one of the advantages of stratified sampling: You can use strata of different sizes in order to obtain the data you need and to allow for differences in the costs of data collection among the different strata. (This last issue does not ordinarily arise in hospital settings.)

Sources of Data

All information is fair game when collecting the data needed to carry out an honest review of the quality of patient care. A decade ago some hospital staff members expressed misgivings with reference to the privacy of the patient and the confidentiality of hospital data. Experience with quality evaluation studies has shown no evidence of violations of privacy and confidentiality in the course of collecting data for such reviews.

The Medical Record

The medical record—either the open chart at the nursing station or zone or the completed record in the medical record department—is the primary source of clinical data. The completed medical record, a most important part of the hospital's data base, is made up of the following components, which are organized into sections by the medical record department.

1. A face sheet, showing admitting office information, including the complete patient identification; the sources of payment; the responsible practitioner; the admitting diagnosis; the primary discharge diagnosis; any invasive diagnostic procedures and any surgery performed on this admission; secondary diagnoses, including preexisting medical problems; and any complications that developed during this hospitalization.

The admission and payment information and identifications are contributed by the admitting office; the clinical information is written by the attending physician. The diagnoses and procedures that are reported by the physician are coded according to the "international classification of diseases" by code clerks in the medical record department. The version of the coding system that is currently in use is called ICD 9CM.

The accurate and complete coding of records is absolutely essential for the description and analysis of the hospital's patient data base.

2. A clinical resume, showing, for this hospitalization, the admitting diagnosis, the diagnostic studies performed, the findings, the treatment employed, any complications or side effects that arose, the progress shown by the patient, the patient's condition at the time of discharge, any medications ordered for posthospital use, instructions given to the patient for his posthospital care, and the final discharge diagnoses.

The clinical resume is written or dictated for transcription by the responsible practitioner or by his authorized designee, such as a house staff member. It must always be signed or countersigned by the responsible practitioner. It is vital, in the interest of efficient data retrieval as well as continuity of care, that the clinical resume be complete and clearly formulated.

3. Reports of the physical examination and relevant medical history at the time of admission. These may be written by the attending physician or by a house staff member acting for him, but they must be signed or countersigned by the responsible practitioner.

4. Orders written by the responsible practitioner for tests, treatments, medications, diet, and so forth. This includes requests for consultations as well.

5. Progress notes written by the attending practitioner and house staff or consultants who see the patient. Such notes should be informative and should reflect the patient's condition. As the Joint Commission repeatedly emphasizes, a progress note should contain more information than "no change" or "improved." Progress notes should occur with sufficient frequency to indicate that this patient is indeed being seen regularly—at least once in each 24 hour period—by the responsible practitioner or his associates.

6. Reports of consultants, if consultations have been requested.

7. A complete report on any operations performed, written

or dictated by the operating surgeon. This report should include the preoperative diagnosis, descriptions of the procedures performed, descriptions of the condition of the tissues, the surgeon's findings, the patient's condition at the end of the procedure, and the postoperative diagnosis.

8. Where surgery has been performed, a complete anesthesia report, showing details of the anesthesia as well as a record of blood transfusions and intravenous therapy.

9. Where surgery has been performed, preanesthesia and postanesthesia evaluation notes, written by a physician or, in the case of a dental procedure, by a qualified oral surgeon.

10. A complete report of any invasive diagnostic procedures, written or dictated by the practitioner who performed the procedure.

11. The preliminary assessment of the patient and a preliminary determination of the level of care required, written by the nurse at the time of admission. Any special protective measures that are needed, such as raised side rails on the bed, are recorded here.

12. The nursing care plan developed for the patient shortly after admission. In this plan the nurses indicate any special tasks that will be carried out for this patient and the schedule to be observed in performing them.

13. The nurses' graphic notes, medication records, intravenous administration records, and any other records of evaluations or treatments that are performed with the nurses' participation. The graphic chart shows the daily record of the patient's vital signs: temperature, pulse, and respirations. In addition this chart shows scheduled blood pressure readings for certain patients. For patients on intravenous hydration, records of intake and output are maintained. Blood transfusion and hyperalimentation charts are maintained by the nurses on an ongoing basis.

14. The nurses' narrative notes from each shift. In these notes the nurses provide a history of the patient's status at specified times and record any treatments given or events that occurred with respect to the patient's condition and progress.

15. Reports showing assessment and treatments by such services as physical therapy and respiratory therapy. These reports should include material showing the patient's condition and progress.

16.   Reports of clinical laboratory tests.

17.   Reports of examinations by the radiology, cardiographic, nuclear medicine, electroencephalographic, or other specialized diagnostic services.

18.   Copies of requisitions for tests, medications, blood, and materials used in the patient's care.

19.   Copies of any forms used by the responsible practitioners and the nursing service in giving the patient instructions for his posthospital care and in indicating the need for a follow-up visit to his physician where this is appropriate.

20.   Signed consents for treatment, any surgery, and any invasive procedures that may take place.

21.   Brief summary of discharge plans.

An enormous amount of data is contained in a completed medical record. Unfortunately, in an effort to perform quality assurance evaluation research during the past 10 years, it has been found that much of the data in these records is of very poor quality. In this respect it appears that the concerns displayed by the American College of Surgeons in 1914 are still justified today.

In identifying the charts that are to be included in a concurrent or retrospective review of the treatment given in connection with a specified diagnosis or operation, the investigator must be able to rely on the accuracy of the label given to the admitting diagnosis, the operation, or the primary discharge diagnosis. It is the primary discharge diagnosis or the operation label that classifies the patient and his admission for all future identification purposes.

If the study involves the collection of data from current charts, the effect of errors in recording the admitting diagnosis is not extremely serious. This is because the reviewer has an opportunity to screen the chart and to identify the actual working diagnosis on the basis of other reports. Furthermore, it is not always possible for the responsible practitioner to state the diagnosis with great precision before diagnostic studies have been performed.

However, the problem of inaccuracy in providing the final label on the record of a discharged patient is far more serious and is actually very common.

In processing the records of discharged patients, the medical record department's code clerk reads what the responsible practitioner has written on the face sheet and defines that patient and his admission in terms of the ICD 9 code that matches the label supplied. From that point on, that admission goes into the hospital's data base for financial and other planning activities under that code.

This problem of data quality is mentioned here because the presence of flawed data makes any evaluation research effort difficult and the findings potentially inaccurate or unrealistic. In addition to the implications for patient care review, a poor data base can have serious consequences for the hospital's financial condition. Where as many as 20 percent of a hospital's discharged patients have been indexed on the basis of inaccurate medical classification—which is often the case—the hospital's case mix analyses, corporate planning studies, and marketing projections cannot be valid.

Nonetheless, with these reservations in mind, the medical record remains a valuable source of data in quality evaluation, particularly of data reflecting clinical events and outcomes.

Utilization Review Records

Although Medicare reimbursement is no longer tied to specified limits on length of stay, hospitals will continue to monitor length of stay in the interest of cost containment. The accreditation standards of the Joint Commission continue to require that hospitals provide for the appropriate allocation of their resources in part by conducting utilization review programs.

Utilization review records are excellent sources of information concerning such elements as the absence of preadmission testing in elective surgery, unjustifiable admissions, the inappropriate or excessive utilization of treatment modalities, and delays in discharge resulting from the occurrence of hospital-generated complications.

Incident Reports

Routine reading of hospital incident reports should be coupled with an effort to keep abreast of the current malpractice literature found in the various health law journals. If the investigator is sensitized to the current malpractice issues and the type of event that often generates a claim, he or she is in a position to identify those situations or events in his or her own hospital that may call for assessment and corrective action as a preventive measure.

In addition to pointing to potential malpractice exposure, incident reports often help to identify hazards to employees or visitors. Where patterns are detected, an assessment is required to bring the situation to the attention of those who can take corrective action in enough time to prevent an accident and a claim.

One method of flagging undesirable events is the use of the so-called morbidity screen. In this process a monthly list is prepared of patients who exhibited certain specified indicators of possible complications of care. The screen's preestablished indicators include such occurrences as a return to the operating room following surgery, the need for ventilatory assistance in the recovery room, excessive length of stay in the recovery room, wound infections, and drug and transfusion reactions.

Department Records

Records of clinical, ancillary, and environmental departments and services are also valuable sources of data. There is one serious problem in using the records of such departments as physical and respiratory therapy in conjunction with medical records. This is the all-too-common observation that these and other ancillary services do not identify and file treatment records by the medical record numbers. This results in delays and excessive labor costs in cross-referencing the patients' records for retrieval.

Records from physical therapy, respiratory therapy, housekeeping, laundry, dietetic, and plant maintenance services are useful in studying problems in infection control. In any study of hospital safety, the preventive maintenance records of such services as radiology, clinical laboratories, pathology, laundry, and building maintenance should be used. When monitoring safety, the reviewer should include the maintenance records of electrically operated beds and other devices used in patient care.

The review of patient billing records for denial of insurance claims or reimbursement is useful in evaluating the quality of medical record data as well as in evaluating the appropriateness of utilization patterns. Records of the social service department contain information that relates to the effectiveness of discharge planning and, in many hospitals, to the way in which follow-up care is organized. Pharmacy records include patient medication profiles that are invaluable in collecting data for studies of antibiotic utilization. Records of surgical suite requisitions for antibiotic preparations to be used in irrigating wounds should be included in monitoring the use of antibiotics.

A great deal of information on case mix can be retrieved from the medical staff admissions profiles that are maintained in many hospitals.

Interview and Observation

In collecting information about many types of performance, the most practical approach is to interview those who perform the tasks in question or to observe them as they work. This approach is particularly useful in assessing the performance of certain housekeeping and maintenance tasks, such as washing corridor floors or dusting the horizontal surfaces in a patient's room. In many evaluation projects in the field of housekeeping and building maintenance, there is no substitute for direct inspection that is carefully documented with reference to preestablished performance criteria.

Many procedures that depend on the manual skills of the performer for effectivness must be observed by someone who is skilled in that task in order to be monitored. An example would be the insertion of an intravenous or Foley catheter. Tasks that involve a series of actions that are not individually documented may also have to be observed if their performance is to be evaluated.

7

Evaluation Research in the Program: Criteria, Data, and the Research Report

The discussion of criteria, data collection and report preparation follows the evaluation research outline shown in Chapter 5.

Criteria

In conducting any type of performance review, whether concurrent or retrospective, it is absolutely essential to apply preestablished written evaluation criteria.

There are three basic types of criteria: structural criteria, process or procedural criteria, and outcome or result criteria.

The structural criteria relate to an organization and the way in which it is put together in order to accomplish its aims. They deal with such matters as governance, management, supervisory channels, the reporting paths, the budget, and the qualifications of the members of the organization. In the hospital the patients are also members of the organization and as such are affected by certain criteria. These criteria address such matters as indications for admission or for admission to a certain special care unit. The patient has to meet these criteria in order to get into the organization.

In evaluating any sort of organization, structural criteria are essential. If the organization itself is not built in such a way as to mobilize the power it needs in order to attain its ends and to guide its members, then the organization cannot function effectively and will probably never reach its goals.

Since structural criteria concern aspects of an organization that are usually matters of record, such as the governing body's bylaws, the licensure of nurses, or the classification of the emergency room, it is easy to detect departures from them. This is the principal reason for the Joint Commission's original reliance upon them.

In 1953, when it assumed the responsibility for surveying the hospitals of the United States and, for a time, of Canada, the Joint Commission was seriously understaffed to perform the job it had undertaken. The new Joint Commission was operating with a field staff whose members represented three of the five member organizations—the American College of Surgeons, the American Medical Association, and the American Hospital Association. The largest group, consisting of eight physicians, represented the American Medical Association and combined their JCAH surveying with their regular AMA review of hospital internship and residency programs. The total number of surveyors available at any given time was 16. These surveyors were physicians and hospital administrators who were salaried employees of their respective professional organizations. Not until January 1964 did the Joint Commission begin to charge hospitals for surveys and assume responsibility for its surveyor payroll.

In the March 1953 Bulletin of the Joint Commission, the director, Dr. Edwin L. Crosby, reported that during January and February of that year 182 hospitals had been surveyed and that plans called for the surveys of 200 more hospitals by the end of the year.[7] By March 1955 the field staff had grown to 20 in the United States and 2 in Canada, but the backlog of hospitals that were overdue for survey had reached 1,295.[8]

A professional evaluating body faced with a workload of these dimensions has time to study only the most visible characteristics of the organizations that it surveys. The Joint Commission was forced to rely on structural criteria that could be documented and that would lend themselves, it was hoped, to uniform interpretation by the various surveyors.

The structural emphasis is seen throughout the standards. For example, the JCAH holds that a hospital must have a governing body of some sort to establish policy and provide general direction. Medical staff members must be qualified to practice their respective professions. The director of nursing must be a registered professional nurse. The organization must have a budget and an annual audit. The emergency room must not be used for performing surgery that should be done in an operating room.

Under the circumstances, developing sound structural standards is the best that an organization like the JCAH can do. It would be impossible for the JCAH surveyors to probe deeply enough into a hospital's activities during an accreditation survey to make supportable judgments about the everyday compliance of its personnel with other types of criteria.

In an effort to respond to the needs of the evaluation of patient care as an activity, a new structural requirement—that the hospital monitor its own performance—was adopted in 1974. In order to comply with the quality assurance requirements, the hospital's personnel would formulate and apply process and outcome criteria.

Process criteria address matters of procedure, method, and technique. Members of professional and technical occupations have always relied on the evaluation of technique to guide them in their performance and in judging the ability of their peers. Process criteria can be very useful in the hands of those who understand the functions being evaluated.

Examples of process criteria can often be found in studies designed by members of technical groups. In the management of fetal distress, the criteria include reference to specific steps, including checking the response of the fetal heart rate to changes in the mother's position every five minutes and the administration of oxygen to the mother at five to six liters per minute. The procedure manuals written by members of services and units in the hospital are excellent sources of process criteria for use in concurrent monitoring.

The difficulty here is that although all the correct procedures may have been performed by fully qualified personnel, the end result may not be consistent with the expectations or plans. Thorough evaluation requires the application of more than structural and process criteria.

This leads us to a consideration of outcome or result criteria. These are criteria that even a layman can usually understand, and therein lies their great value.

Examples of outcome criteria include the following:

- A wound infection rate below 5 percent of all operations performed during a year.
- A Medicare claims denial rate of less than 8 percent of all claims submitted.
- An average length of stay for unilateral inguinal herniorrhaphy of no more than 4 days for patients aged 16 to 64.
- A rate of returned, misdirected trays of less than 4 percent of trays prepared.

You could say that these outcome criteria represent the goals of good hospital care and efficient hospital management—the two are not mutually exclusive. As the investigator, you can use an outcome criterion in your study. Then, in those cases in which the outcome criterion is not met, you can ask, with Codman, "If not, why not?" One way of identifying the reasons for failure to meet the outcome criterion is to employ the process criteria formulated by the professional, technical, and administrative personnel who are familiar with the various clinical, fiscal, or environmental functions involved in the study.

All three kinds of criteria—structural, process, and outcome— are useful in conducting evaluation studies. None of them should be ignored. If you find a pattern of failure to comply with an outcome criterion, look for the structural-organizational or process factors that may have contributed to the unfavorable results.

Before beginning the collection of data, obtain the relevant criteria from the staff of the service involved in the study. The investigator should be ready to edit or rewrite the criteria to make them as precise and as clear as possible to an individual who is not acquainted with the technical aspects of the functions under review.

One important reason for writing the criteria is to enable those who are trained in data collection to detect variations from the criteria when these turn up in the data. Another important reason is to forestall complaints of unfairness from any service or individual whose performance fails to meet one or more of the criteria.

In writing criteria of any kind, avoid ambiguity. Never use vague terms that may be subject to varying interpretations. Avoid using words like *satisfactory, adequate, plentiful,* and *normal.* Interpretations of what is normal vary from one expert to another. When a numerical value is involved, as in a temperature or blood pressure reading, insist that the clinical experts give you the exact value or range of values they have in mind.

Here are a few examples of common flaws in the framing of criteria:

- Patients treated for viral hepatitis

Poor Language: At discharge, condition improved.

Question: How is the nonmedically trained data collector to know what is meant by "improved"?

Better Language: At discharge, presenting signs and symptoms, such as jaundice, absent or ameliorated.

- Patients having below-knee amputation

Poor Language: Preoperatively, patient given postoperative instructions.

Question: How will a data collector who is not a member of the nursing service know what these instructions are?

Better Language: Preoperatively, patient given instructions as to positioning in bed, use of trapeze, body image and phantom pain, and postanesthesia deep breathing and coughing.

- Patients with carcinoma of the lung

Poor Language: In the chart prior to surgery, documentation of evidence of lung tumor.

Question: How will the data collector identify such evidence when he finds it?

Better Language: In the chart prior to surgery, documentation of either X-ray or bronchoscopic evidence of lung tumor or positive sputum cytology report.

Sometimes your experts will give you a criterion of good practice in their discipline and then engage in a heated and highly technical discussion of all the cases in which this criterion would not apply. They're telling you that there are exceptions to the criterion—that's manageable. Simply record the criterion and the exceptions for your own guidance in gathering data. Use a form like this:

CRITERION: Upper gastrointestinal tract X-rays performed.

Exceptions:

UGI performed within past three months and documented in record.

Endoscopy revealing duodenal or peptic ulcer done prior to UGI.

Patient taken to surgery before UGI could be performed.

Not all criteria must be stated in positive terms. The experts may wish to ensure that some particular procedure that should not be performed for the patient group being studied is discovered if it occurs in the course of the study. In other words, they may be concerned about some procedure that is often contraindicated for these patients, and they want to be sure that its occurrence is noted and documented. This criterion can be stated in this rather convoluted style:

CRITERION: Absence of XYZ procedure.

Actually, most data collectors in health care facilities simply use the 100 percent (present) and 0 percent (absent) convention to indicate the criteria that should be found and those that should be absent from the records being studied.

It is easy to handle the situation in which a particular patient care procedure is usually contraindicated but indicated under specific circumstances. For this situation, assign the procedure a zero standard (0 percent) and list the exceptions—the exceptions are the indications.

Label those criteria that should be found in the data source with an identification that is convenient for you, such as "100 percent" or "present." Label those that should not be found with "0 percent" or "absent." The expression "100 percent" does not mean that the attribute should be present in 100 percent of the cases. The expressions "100 percent" and "0 percent" are merely intended to indicate the presence or absence of the attributes listed in the criteria. Examples of model sets of criteria are shown in Appendixes 1 and 2.

Collection and Analysis of Data

Concurrent data collecting is emphasized here on three grounds. One is the importance of identifying malpractice exposure before any serious consequences have occurred. Second, from the standpoint of minimizing hospital expense it is essential to identify inefficient utilization patterns promptly. Finally, in connection with its quality assurance standard, the Joint Commission is focusing primarily on concurrent monitoring of care.

For some purposes, such as identifying and documenting behavioral patterns believed to have a bearing on poor outcomes, retrospective review continues to be useful. However, it is no longer the principal type of evaluation exercise that it was several years ago.

Concurrent monitoring does not necessarily mean that data on a given subject are collected for 365 days every year. The collection of information is meaningless unless at some point the information is analyzed and used to develop some conclusions. Therefore, a study involving concurrent monitoring of a set of behaviors should be designed to include provisions for the analysis of the data that are available at a given point and for the preparation of a report. At that time, data collection on that subject should be suspended pending the outcome of the analysis.

The time frame for data collection depends on the incidence of the attribute in the study population or the frequency with which the event under study occurs. It may take six months to collect useful data on phototherapy in hyperbilirubinemia in a small community hospital. In a medical center with an average daily census of 700 patients, however, one week may be ample time for a concurrent investigation of the reasons for the inability of the pharmacy to deliver medications to the correct nursing stations in a timely manner.

Accountants' columnar pads are extremely useful for recording data. The page can be set up as a worksheet with the criteria coded by number, usually at the head of each column to be used.

The numbers identifying the cases being studied can be recorded as the row numbers. This type of data display form makes it easy to summarize the available information at any time and to prepare a report on short notice. This is far more efficient than using individual case sheets for recording data.

The analysis of data in quality monitoring or review should be kept simple. The result should be a summary, in absolute and percentage terms, of the performance with reference to each criterion. This can be expressed in either of two ways:

- The number of cases (events or patients) that met each criterion.
- The number of cases in which each criterion was not met.

The fundamental technique used is the frequency distribution. This approach usually satisfies the requirements in terms of pointing to patterns of variation from accepted policy and procedure as these are reflected in criteria. Any patterns of consistent, repeated variation from a particular criterion should be analyzed with reference to the structural factors involved, such as the identified unit, practitioners, shift, or day of the week.

Where patterns of association appear among the variations, an inquiry should be made into the possibility of interdependence. These possibilities can usually be explored without using any techniques of statistical inference. However, it may be impossible, because of the large numbers of practitioners involved or for some other reason, to obtain the needed information by means of interviewing or some other direct method. Where this is the case and further analysis appears warranted, one of the common nonparametric tests of association should be employed. This approach is unnecessary in most hospital quality assurance research.

In terms of the evaluation research outline in Chapter 5, the next step in the process is the preparation of the research report.

The Research Report

Even in a system that emphasizes concurrent monitoring, it is necessary from time to time to pull the findings together in a report. This step enables the services that were reviewed to document the results and to plan any necessary corrective actions. Quality review reports that also reflect utilization and risk exposure are required for decision-making purposes by the governing body, the administration, and the medical staff.

Evaluation reports dealing with a service or department within the administrative organization should be reviewed by the director of standards along with the head of the service and the service liaison representative. Evaluation reports concerning the medical staff or any of its members should be reviewed with the relevant chief of service and the medical staff liaison representative before being submitted to the medical staff executive committee.

Reports should be kept as brief and as simple as possible. This can be done without disregarding any essential information. Such a report can be outlined as follows:

SAMPLE OUTLINE FOR EVALUATION RESEARCH REPORT

Name of Service, Department, or Unit Reviewed

1. Subject or activity reviewed or monitored
2. Reason for this research with reference to any of the following that may be applicable:
   a. Routine medical staff review in compliance with provisions of quality assurance plan
   b. Investigation of possible problem in patient care, specifically defined
   c. Risk and malpractice exposure
   d. Enhancement of claims reimbursement
   e. Case mix management and DRG analysis
   f. Utilization pattern analysis
   g. Unit productivity
   h. Other issues involved
3. Study sample
   a. Size of sample
   b. Composition of sample in terms of sex, age, or other attributes used in defining the sample
   c. Time frame defining the sample
4. Evaluation criteria used
5. Data sources used
6. Data collection methods used, with the time period during which the data were collected
7. Summary of the findings, including any of the following that may be applicable:
   a. Frequency distributions and percentage compliance with each criterion

SAMPLE OUTLINE *(continued)*

    b. Histograms or bar charts
    c. Simple graphs showing any patterns found
8. Brief narrative summary with interpretation and any recommendations of the director of standards
9. The scheduled date on which a follow-up evaluation will be reported, if this action appears justified by the findings.

The periodic reports prepared for the medical staff in compliance with the JCAH standards on medical staff activities should follow essentially the same outline form.

An example of an evaluation research report can be found in Appendix 3.

8

The Quality Assurance Program: Corrective Action, Follow-Up, and Program Evaluation

Corrective Action

Responsibility for Corrective Action

The basic premise underlying the model that was developed in the last four chapters is that responsibility for conducting all of the quality review and monitoring in the hospital is vested in a central office of standards, which is a unit within the corporate organization. The fundamental responsibility of this office is the administration of the hospital's policies in quality assurance, risk control, and utilization control.

Another premise is that, with two exceptions, there are no committees functioning within the structure of the program. The two exceptions are the quality assurance, risk control, and utilization control committee of the governing body and the credentials committee of the medical staff.

The function of the governing body committee is to develop policy and to provide oversight and general direction to the

program. The function of the credentials committee is to fulfill
the medical staff's responsibility to evaluate candidates for
medical staff appointment and reappointment and to submit
recommendations to the governing body, through the medical staff
executive committee, concerning medical staff appointment,
reappointment, and privileges.

This allocation of responsibility and authority is emphasized
here because of the need to develop organizational strategies to
overcome the paralysis that characterizes the hospital administration's approach to corrective action. Under the common committee
structure it has been too easy to shift the responsibility for taking
remedial measures from one committee to another.

The ultimate responsibility and authority for corrective action
lies with the hospital's governing body. The only authority
exercised by the medical staff in this area is that which is related
to the very membership of a practitioner in the group, to the
scope of his clinical privileges, and to his admitting privileges. It
has no authority to recommend any sanctions other than the
extremely severe ones previously described. As mentioned earlier
the severity of the credentials committee's sanctions makes them
inappropriate for use in most situations calling for corrective
action.

Since the governing body can receive and consider only those
reports and recommendations that are submitted to it, it has been
hampered in carrying out its responsibility to improve the quality
of hospital care. It receives from the medical staff only those
recommendations that address such matters as appointment,
reappointment, and the delineation, restriction, or termination of
privileges with respect to quality assurance.

It is necessary to devise a plan whereby the hospital's administration can exercise a more active and timely direction over
matters of quality assurance, risk control, and utilization, including many that affect the medical staff.

Certainly the present role and mission of the medical staff
credentials committee should be preserved. However, it must also
be recognized that there is more to medical staff quality evaluation
and maintenance than the credentialling process. Therefore,
responsibility and authority for developing plans for corrective
action outside the purview of the credentials committee should be
vested in a corporate staff member who is accountable to the

corporation, such as the director of the corporate office of standards.

The Plan for Corrective Action

Defining the Nature of the Deviations from Criteria. Assume that the report of a monitoring study has revealed deviations from the criteria that are significant in terms of extent; potential hazards to patient, staff, or visitor welfare; or some combination of these. Such a finding points to the need for some sort of corrective action.

The dimensions of good or high performance are already known, because these were incorporated in the evaluation criteria applied in the study. The objective of the exercise is to bring about conformity with the high level of performance as this is defined in the evaluation criteria. The effort to achieve a high performance level will require some change in the procedures employed. It may be that the procedural criteria applied were entirely appropriate but not observed. Conversely it could be that the prescribed procedures, although they were followed, were not adequate to bring about the desired outcomes.

Carrying Out Corrective Action. In either case it is necessary to decide which steps will be taken to bring about conformity with the definition of high performance. Assuming that the staff of the office of standards is performing the analytical and planning work, all decisions regarding technical and clinical technique must be discussed with and approved by professional staff members of the service or department involved. The steps agreed on should be listed in a memorandum to be signed by a representative of the office of standards and a representative of the service or department involved.

Once the necessary changes have been agreed on, the next step is to assign the administrative responsibility for implementing these changes. Where the problem involves two or more services, it would be appropriate to set up a task force including the heads of the services involved. Where the problem involves only one service, the head of that service should carry out the necessary changes.

A schedule for the implementation of each step and for completion of the project should be established. The degree of complexity in this schedule depends on the nature of the corrective action plan. If the corrective action project is going to be lengthy and complex, involving input from several different sources, it may be appropriate to set up a Gantt chart schedule form or to set up a critical path management plan. If this is the case the development of the schedule is a responsibility of the office of standards. Examples of appropriate Gantt charts and critical path management plans are shown in Appendixes 4 and 5.

Where the corrective action involves only one or a few administrative decisions and explanations on the part of a department head, all that is needed is a target date for completion. Experience shows that the latter situation is far more common than the former.

In the course of implementing the action plan, the role of the director of standards is to monitor progress with reference to the schedule and to prepare a final report. This completion report will vary from a one-paragraph memorandum for the file to a comprehensive summary intended for review by the chief executive officer. Its format and content will depend on the gravity of the situation that has been corrected and the complexity of the corrective action. Each hospital's administration will develop its own guidelines for the documentation of corrective action.

The Change Apparatus in the Administrative Organization

The hospital's administrative organization is already set up to facilitate the implementation of necessary corrective action projects. In most cases it has relatively clear channels of authority and supervision and is supported by a system of rewards and sanctions. The mechanisms for modifying behavior in the interest of quality assurance exist in the form of the organization's personnel evaluation system.

In order to utilize the existing system, it is essential that relevant information that is generated in the course of departmental quality monitoring or reviews be made available to those who supervise department heads. While quality assurance records should not be filed in the personnel department, the individual responsible for assessing the performance of a department head should be encouraged to review the summary reports on any relevant quality evaluation studies. This should be done in the office of standards at the time of the department head's routine annual performance evaluation. The department head's record in meeting the hospital's quality assurance standards and objectives should be given as much weight as the other dimensions of his or her performance.

The Change Apparatus of the Medical Staff

Medical Staff Bylaws

Any effort on the part of the governing body, the medical staff leadership, or the administration to bring about behavioral change in the medical staff is hampered by the punitive character of the suspension provisions of medical staff bylaws. Because of this, definitive action is usually not taken until a catastrophic situation has arisen. There is no provision in the bylaws for timely and effective preventive action of a nonpunitive nature. This void could be filled by including references to the hospital's quality assurance, risk control, and utilization control mechanism in the bylaws.

Problems exist in applying the corrective action provisions of the medical staff bylaws in quality assurance matters. One of these is the fact that they include no direct reference to the obligation of the medical staff member to comply with the requirements of the hospital's quality assurance, risk control, and utilization review program. It should be made clear that compliance with the bylaws includes compliance with the hospital's policies in the areas of quality, risk, and utilization. A provision identifying adherence to these policies as one of the specific responsibilities of medical staff membership should be added to the medical staff bylaws, rules, and regulations.

Medical staff bylaws typically contain lists of the factors that will be considered by the credentials committee in its review of applications at reappointment time. These lists usually include references to such things as attendance at meetings, participation in medical staff affairs, general attitude toward practice, and the practitioner's health status. To these lists should be added a requirement of adherence to hospital policies on quality assurance and utilization control. It is unnecessary to mention risk control in the lists, because that factor is logically subsumed under quality control.

In applying for appointment or reappointment to the staff, the practitioner acknowledges that he has read and subscribes to the bylaws, rules, and regulations. He makes a commitment to comply with the provisions of those documents and to carry out the responsibilities of staff membership. In the interest of clarifying medical staff commitment to the hospital's quality, risk, and utilization control policies, it is vital that the bylaws contain explicit reference to the policies and to the combined program.

Medical staff bylaws must be consistent with the policies and bylaws of the governing body. They cannot be revised or adopted without the approval of the governing body. The governing body has the authority to require that the medical staff bylaws contain adequate provisions for ensuring medical staff compliance with hospital policies and programs in quality, risk, and utilization control. It is the responsibility of the governing body to exercise its authority in this area. Since Joint Commission accreditation requirements call for periodic review of governing body and medical staff bylaws, the appropriate revisions can be made at the time of such review. At that time the governing body can withhold its approval of a set of bylaws that do not contain the relevant provisions.

Techniques for Facilitating Change

When the appropriate bylaw provisions have been made, providing the structural framework to authorize corrective action, a variety of management techniques can be put into action. The application of any of these measures is stimulated by the information that is generated through the evaluation system. The information, the nature of which will be discussed later, is transmitted by the office of standards to the medical staff liaison representative in the routine and special evaluation reports. The role of the medical staff liaison representative is to confer with the relevant service chief and the hospital's medical director, if there is one, in order to decide on the most appropriate and effective measures to take.

Traditionally, it was generally believed that requiring continuing education programs for the medical staff was the solution. This has been shown to be erroneous. Very few deviations from criteria of good practice are the result of ignorance on the part of the practitioner. In addition it is hardly cost-effective to mount expensive educational programs addressed to the entire staff in order to retrain one or a few individuals. The months of preparation needed to secure a speaker and to plan a program cause delays in the correction of a potentially serious problem. Finally, it has often been observed by medical staff members who faithfully participate in their hospitals' educational programs that the very members they consider most in need of updating and of intellectual stimulation are the ones who consistently fail to attend.

The consultative, nonpunitive, face-to-face discussion for the purpose of exploring patient care problems and developing solutions has been successfully employed in a number of hospitals. In terms of the model being developed here, the participants are the chief of the service to which the affected practitioner belongs, the director of standards, and the practitioner. The role of the director of standards is to respond to questions, to explain the details of the evaluation research that generated recommendations, and to clarify governing body and hospital policy if necessary.

The service chief may, following his evaluation of the circumstances, conclude that there is no reason for the service to recommend any change in the practitioner's patient care. Where the service concludes that a change is in order, the chief transmits his recommendations to the practitioner by means of a memorandum—with a copy sent to the director of standards. The issues of file maintenance, privacy, and confidentiality are discussed later.

Where the service has recommended a change it should reinforce its recommendation by informing the practitioner that his work will be individually monitored for a stated period—six months, for example—with particular attention being focused on the problem that has been revealed. In many such situations the service also requires that the practitioner obtain consultation in specified areas of patient care. Where the problem involves surgery, the service often requires during the monitoring period that the practitioner arrange to have another member of the surgical attending staff scrubbed and present when he performs the type of operation that was under review.

Provision should be made for reevaluation of the practitioner's patient care at the end of the monitoring period. Reference to any requirements imposed on the practitioner, such as those mentioned previously, as well as to the monitoring process should be included in the memorandum from the service chief.

In hospitals where the corrective approach previously described is employed, it is customary to keep all materials related to the process, including notices, memoranda, and monitoring or evaluation reports, in the incident files. No copies of the relevant documents, including the memoranda, are placed in the practitioner's medical staff file. It is probably unnecessary to state that materials reflecting any activities of the quality assurance program are never placed in medical record files or in the files of medical staff members. The identity of the practitioner should be protected by using specially assigned codes for each such occasion. In other words, the practitioner's regularly assigned hospital code number should never be used in monitoring or review reports.

Data for Decision-Making Purposes

A few hospitals have established stable systems for bringing about medical staff corrective action, using procedures very similar to those outlined previously. However, in many hospitals the service chiefs and other medical staff members who are responsible for maintaining high quality in patient care must rely on informal methods of identifying those few practitioners who are in need of consultative assistance. Their situation is a difficult one. They must always avoid becoming involved in real or imagined witch-hunts. They cannot receive practice data on all staff members through the scheduled medical staff reviews on antibiotic use, blood transfusions, and surgical practice, because not all of the staff members use these modalities. Even where the hospital maintains an active program of clinical review studies, any sampling plan may miss the one patient care episode that points to the need for critical study of a practitioner's performance.

Greater use of the medical staff profiles that are now maintained in many hospitals may be of some assistance in gathering practice data. These profiles are data bases usually showing the staff member's case mix, admissions, average length of stay, patient days, and contributions to departmental and hospital revenue over the course of each calendar quarter and year. It is possible to add a few indicators of practice patterns to this data base. For example, the following data, expressed as percentages of the practitioner's annual admissions, would be informative:

• Number of readmissions for same diagnosis within two weeks following discharge from this or another hospital by the same practitioner.

      Name of variable: Early readmission rate.

• Number of cases of length of stay in excess of hospital's maximum for the DRG represented.

      Name of variable: Excess LOS.

• Sample estimate of number of admissions not justified on basis of hospital's admission criteria for the relevant DRG.

      Name of variable: Unjustified admissions.

• Number of Medicare or other third-party payer claims rejected or reduced.

      Name of variable: Rejected claims.

These data should be collected and stored in the medical staff utilization data base or profile material for six months in order to determine the hospitalwide statistical norms to be used in initial comparisons.

When enough information has been stored to permit the calculation of hospital mean values, the relevant standard deviation for each value should be calculated, and a range of acceptable values established for each of the variables. These ranges are defined as the group norms to stand until the profiles are updated. Each time the entire data base is updated according to the schedule established by the business office or the management information service, the amount of each medical staff member's variation from the current group norm on each variable should be calculated and reported.

Periodic reviews of the variations from group norms can be conducted by the office of standards in order to identify patterns of practice that could be associated with inappropriate admissions, prolonged morbidity, the occurrence of complications prolonging hospital stays, premature discharge of patients, or the inefficient utilization of hospital resources.

The statistical data do not constitute definitive findings of any kind. They would be used merely as indicators calling attention to patterns that may or may not reflect inadequate patient care. In each case a study of the practice involved, designed as a retrospective or concurrent review with the use of preestablished criteria and an appropriate sample, would be required.

Similarly, the periodic reviews of the use of antibiotics and blood as well as the surgical case review performed for the medical staff should be analyzed by the office of standards for statistical indicators of practice patterns that are not consistent with medical staff criteria. Patterns of unjustified variation from the criteria call for further investigation on either a concurrent or retrospective basis. In any such studies, the use of preestablished written criteria and adequate sampling are essential.

This approach is based on the use of hard data and peer comparison. It is a defensible way to initiate the review of a given practice in the presence of evidence suggesting that a review may be indicated.

The corrective action methods described would be supported by the two elements needed to legitimize such efforts: bylaw provisions specifying adherence to the hospital's quality assurance standards as a responsibility of the medical staff member and the use of objective, uniformly applied criteria in selecting practice patterns for detailed study. With this sort of approach, the service chief and medical staff officers are not placed in an untenable position in carrying out their responsibilities.

The Follow-Up Review

Where the original study of the performance of a service or of the practice pattern of a medical staff member resulted in findings of significant, unjustified variations from criteria, the corrective action plan should specify a time period during which improvement in performance is expected to take place.

The length of this time period will vary depending on the nature and complexity of the corrections to be made. If the retraining of personnel or the revision of procedures is necessary, it is important to allow enough time for the personnel involved to benefit from the training or to adapt to the new procedures. If two or more services are involved, more time is usually needed than if only one service must make changes. If the recommendations for change involve the purchase of equipment, adequate lead time must be allowed for ordering, delivery, installation, and training.

In cases involving medical staff members, the time period before the initiation of a follow-up study varies inversely with the severity of the potential impact of the observed deficiency on patient care and with the incidence of the diagnostic entity in the staff member's practice. The length of time should be determined by the chief of the service on the basis of his clinical expertise and his knowledge of the practitioner's patient mix. Where ongoing monitoring of a practitioner's patient care is employed, periods of three or six months are commonly specified.

At the end of the prescribed time the office of standards performs a follow-up study. This study is addressed only to the criteria in which deficiencies occurred.

If the office of standards determines that performance has improved and meets or approaches hospital criteria, a brief report documenting this finding is written. This concludes the review—at least for the time being.

If it is determined that performance of a unit of the administrative organization continues to fall below hospital criteria, this finding is reported to the operating executive to whom the head of the unit reports. From then on the matter goes through the administrative system and is handled as is any other example of inadequate supervisory performance.

If a follow-up study reveals the continued failure of a medical staff member to comply with the hospital's criteria, this finding is reported to the relevant service chief, to the medical director, if there is one, and to the president of the staff.

It is assumed that the bylaws clearly state the obligation of staff members to meet the medical staff criteria of patient care. The affected practitioner was warned of the need for improvement and was given an opportunity to change his practice patterns to comply with the guidelines laid down by his clinical service. In the face of his failure to respond, the medical staff is required to fulfill its responsibility to the governing body by taking appropriate action to protect the hospital's level of patient care.

The service that is affected can refer the matter to the executive committee with a recommendation for the restriction or suspension of privileges in the interest of good patient care. If he chooses, the affected practitioner can avail himself of the appeals procedure provided for in the bylaws. In any event the presence of bylaws recognition of the quality assurance requirements and of the documented performance evaluation will support the service's recommendations for corrective action.

Program Evaluation

There are at least two sound reasons for an annual formal evaluation of the effectiveness of the hospital's combined standards program. First, there is the need for an administrative assessment of the program's cost-effectiveness and productivity in terms of implementing hospital policy. Second, the Joint Commission requires that the quality assurance program be evaluated at least annually.

Evaluating the effectiveness of a quality assurance program in improving patient care entails developing criteria. In terms of the JCAH guidelines, the hospital should be able to demonstrate that its program is "ongoing, comprehensive, effective in improving patient care/clinical performance and conducted with cost-efficiency."[9] Variables reflecting these criteria can be developed as follows:

Ongoing Character of the Program

That the program is ongoing rather than sporadically implemented can be shown by means of the annual and quarterly schedules established by the office of standards together with the various units participating in the program. The schedules of monitoring studies, reports, and consultations reflect the continuing nature of the quality assurance effort. These are useful in demonstrating compliance with this requirement to the JCAH Hospital Accreditation Program surveyors at the time of the accreditation survey.

Comprehensive Character of the Program

The establishment of a hospitalwide, centrally administered quality assurance program is clear evidence of the comprehensive coverage of the program's activities. Documentation of this coverage is found in the schedules and review reports referred to previously. The recorded active participation of the medical staff and departmental representatives in the quality assurance plan is additional evidence of the program's comprehensive coverage. A list of the studies and monitoring activities performed should be maintained and periodically updated to provide documentation of the program's coverage.

Effectiveness in Enhancing Patient Care

The effectiveness of the program in enhancing the quality of patient care can also be assessed and documented. One method involves presenting the evidence found in follow-up study reports, whether these are one-paragraph memoranda for the record or more detailed consultative reports describing fairly complicated corrective projects. To provide a measure of success, a running "fulfillment rate"—a simple calculation of the number of resolved problems as a percentage of total follow-up studies—should be maintained by the office of standards. Such a rate can be maintained for each clinical and administrative service in a relatively complex organization.

Other evidence of improvement can take the form of an annual comparison of rates of such events as unjustified admissions, excessive lengths of stay, inappropriate utilization of hospital resources, surgical wound infections, hospital-generated complications, inappropriate utilization of antibiotics and blood, unjustified surgical procedures as determined by the medical staff, and reduction and denial of third-party payer claims. Maintaining these statistics should be one of the routine ongoing responsibilities of the office of standards, so that up-to-date summaries can be prepared each quarter or each year as part of the annual evaluation of the program.

Cost-Efficiency of the Program

In the 1984 version of the interpretations to its quality assurance standard, the Joint Commission continues to specify that the quality assurance program should be "conducted with cost efficiency." This does not mean what you may think.

Although the language suggests that the JCAH wishes to encourage hospitals to conduct their quality assurance activities in a cost-effective manner, it was actually the intent of the commissioners to convey their desire to encourage the cost-effective utilization of patient care services. In other words, it was not the program's cost-effectiveness that was addressed in the interpretation, but the cost-effectiveness of direct patient care.[10]

The favorable impact of the quality assurance activity on the costs of patient care is demonstrated in an analysis of the utilization of hospital resources. Thus where the quality assurance program can be shown to be instrumental in reducing the rates of excessive lengths of stay, unjustified admissions, hospital-generated complications, and inappropriate or excessive resource utilization, it can be argued that the program is operating to reduce or contain the cost of care. Each of these elements contributes to the cost of hospital care without producing any benefit to the patient.

While the statistical record of program fulfillment should be continually maintained, a summary report showing the degree to which the program meets its objectives should be prepared annually. This report is intended for review by the governing body as well as by corporate management and the medical staff. An example of the type of exhibit recommended is included in Appendix 6.

In any evaluation of the entire quality assurance process or of an individual program, it would be desirable to explore program expense. However, it would be unrealistic to make any generalizations about the expense of conducting quality assurance programs in hospitals at this time for the following reasons:

- There is no uniformity in the cost accounting approaches used by hospitals in identifying this area of expense.

- In many hospitals the activity is not identified for budget purposes. Rather, it is carried out through the nursing service or the medical record department with no effort to segregate the expense.

- Even those hospitals that identify the activity for purposes of reporting to the AHA's Hospital Administrative Services program employ different methods of calculating service load.

While direct expenses and salary expenses are reported in the HAS Monitrend Reports, these figures are based on the "discharge unit." Total annual discharge units are calculated as the sum of the following:

Adult discharges.

Nursery discharges.

One third of outpatient visits.

One third of emergency department visits.

The discrepancy occurs in identifying outpatient and emergency department visits. Assume that a given patient visits the outpatient department for four diagnostic studies—an EKG, a chest X-ray, a complete blood count, and a urinalysis—as part of the preadmission screening before elective surgery. In a large medical center this means that he visits three different sections of the outpatient clinic or facility—the cardiology section, the diagnostic radiology section, and the clinical laboratory section. Each of these visits is usually counted separately for a total of three outpatient visits, contrary to AHA instructions.

In some facilities, because it is a separate charge, the urinalysis is also counted as a single visit. Thus the total number of outpatient visits entering into the hospital's statistics is four. In another hospital, where all of the tests and studies may be performed in one section or physical area, the preadmission screening may be counted as one outpatient visit.

In some hospitals tests performed in the emergency room are not counted as separate visits. Thus only a single emergency room visit is reported. In other hospitals, if an emergency room patient is sent to, for example, the radiology section to have an X-ray performed, this is counted as a second visit.

The key to the number of visits that is reported by the hospital is the number of times the patient registers either for a visit or for an individual diagnostic procedure. This varies with the patient flow patterns established by each facility.

The other major factor making reported program expense figures unreliable is the custom in many hospitals of including quality evaluation data gathering, analysis, and report preparation in the regular duties of nursing, medical records, and other

personnel. In many hospitals a significant but largely undocumented number of labor-hours per month are presently spent in
quality assurance planning and reporting meetings. Collecting
data, performing statistical analyses, and writing reports accounts
for an additional number of undocumented labor-hours per month.
In payroll accounting these hours often are categorized as nonpro-
ductive time.

For these reasons it is impossible at this time to place much
credence in published data reflecting the expenses of quality
assurance or patient care evaluation activities on a regional or
national scale. Because of the way in which the "discharge unit"
is calculated, the expense per patient is probably deflated in large
hospitals and medical centers, while it is relatively inflated in
small hospitals. In either case the time spent by professional
health care personnel on the administrative details of quality
monitoring and review is presently not documented adequately for
cost analysis purposes.

Appendixes
Notes
Bibliography
Index

Appendixes

Appendix 1

ANTIBIOTIC USAGE
CLINDAMYCIN (CLEOCIN)

REVIEW

Criterion	Standard (in %)
INDICATIONS FOR THE USE OF CLINDAMYCIN	
1. Presence of a serious anaerobic infection susceptible to Clindamycin or of a serious infection caused by susceptible streptococci, pneumococci, or staphylococci in a patient who cannot take penicillin	100
CLINICAL AND LABORATORY INDICATORS FOR THE USE OF CLINDAMYCIN	
2. Presence of one or more of the following elements:	100

109

Criterion	Standard (in %)

a. Culture showing susceptible organism

b. Fever above 102°F

c. Chest X-ray consistent with bacterial pneumonia, empyema, or lung abscess

d. Tender, hot, swollen, erythematous tissues on physical examination

e. Peritonitis, perforation of a hollow viscus, or intraabdominal abscess

f. Infection clinically present at surgery

g. Contaminated wound

CONTRAINDICATIONS TO THE USE OF CLINDAMYCIN

3. Presence of any of the following elements: 0

a. Nonbacterial infection

b. Allergy to Clindamycin or Lincomycin

c. History of colitis
   Exception: No other appropriate antibiotic available

d. Severe renal or liver disease
   Exception: No other appropriate antibiotic available. Dose to be reduced to 1.2 gm/day.
   Record Analyst: Severe renal disease is reflected in BUN greater than 50, creatinine greater than 5, and creatinine clearance below 10.
   Severe liver disease is reflected in albumin less than 2, bilirubin greater than 10, and SGOT more than 3 times normal.
   Find data in laboratory reports.

e. Severe urinary tract infection

f. Meningitis

g. Pregnancy
   Exception: Presence of life-threatening infection with no other appropriate antibiotic available

h. Concomitant administration of Erythromycin

Criterion	Standard (in %)

LABORATORY STUDIES

4. The following tests and findings:
   a. At least 1 appropriate culture (blood, sputum, vaginal, or wound as applicable) — 100
   b. CBC, differential and urinalysis — 100
   c. Bilirubin less than 10 mg % — 100
   d. Albumin greater than 2 gm % — 100
   e. SGOT less than 3 times normal value — 100
   f. BUN equal to 50 mg/100 ml or less — 100

DOSAGE AND ADMINISTRATION

5. Dose 0.6–2.8 gms/24 hours — 100
   Exception: In presence of liver or renal disease, dose less than 1.2 gms/day
6. Route oral, intravenous, or intramuscular — 100

MANAGEMENT

7. Vital signs, intake and output, and response to Clindamycin monitored and documented — 100
8. Patient monitored for evidence of complications — 100
9. Management of complications
   a. Rash or other allergic reaction attributed to Clindamycin
      Use of Clindamycin stopped — 100
   b. Diarrhea or colitis
      (1) Clindamycin discontinued — 100
      (2) Where diarrhea persists for 48 hours or patient passes blood, proctosigmoidoscopy performed for evaluation — 100

INDICATIONS FOR DISCONTINUATION OF CLINDAMYCIN

10. Presence of any of the following elements: — 100
    a. Temperature below 100°F for 48 hours
    b. Failure of clinical response after 4 days
    c. Culture report showing organism not susceptible to Clindamycin

Appendix 2

PACEMAKER IMPLANTATION

SUGGESTED SAMPLE

Patients whose discharge diagnoses include skin necrosis, hematoma, wound infection, pacemaker malfunction, or pacemaker failure, in association with pacemaker implantation.

REVIEW

Criterion	Standard (in %)
JUSTIFICATION FOR EXTENDED STAY	
1. Presence of skin necrosis, hematoma, wound infection, pacemaker malfunction, or failure following pacemaker implantation	100
PREOPERATIVE STUDY AND CARE	
2. In the chart prior to the implantation,	
a. Documentation of the presence of any one of the following:	100
(1) Acquired complete auriculo-ventricular block	
(2) Sinus node dysfunction	
(3) Intermittent complete heart block (right bundle branch block, left bundle branch block or bifascicular)	
(4) Acute myocardial infarction with anterior wall heart block	
(5) Congenital complete auriculoventricular block or surgical auriculoventricular block with symptoms	
(6) Recurrent ventricular tachycardia	
(7) Atrial fibrillation with slow ventricular rate (paroxysmal atrial tachy-	

Criterion	Standard (in %)
cardia, Wolff-Parkinson-White Syndrome)	
(8) Bradycardia resulting from electrolyte imbalance (hyperkalemia)	
(9) Pacemaker failure	
b. History with specific reference to any of the following:	100
(1) Stokes-Adams attacks	
(2) Syncope and/or dizziness	
(3) Tachycardia	
(4) Bradycardia	
(5) Intractable congestive heart failure	
(6) Hypertensive vascular disease	
c. Physical examination report with findings of either	100
(1) Bradycardia less than 40 per minute, irregular, with EKG evidence of heart block	
(2) Tachycardia greater than 120 per minute not controlled by medication	
3. Laboratory and other studies including	
a. CBC, urinalysis, and admission panel	100
b. Coagulation profile	100
c. Serology	100
d. Chest X-ray	100
e. EKG	100
4. Preoperative nursing care including	
a. Patient assessment including vital signs, brief relevant history, and present complaint	100
b. History of allergies and drug sensitivities	100
c. Formulation of care plan based on assessment and objectives	100
d. Patient orientation to care and planned procedures	100
e. Implementation of appropriate cardiac care plan	100
f. Preoperative instruction and preparation	100

Criterion	Standard (in %)
5. Anesthesiologist's preoperative evaluation of patient with specification of risk level	100

SURGICAL MANAGEMENT

6. Implantation of pacemaker	100
7. X-ray to ascertain correct positioning of pacemaker	100
8. Threshold of pacemaker tested and recorded in room in which implantation is performed **Exception:** Temporary pacemaker	
9. Pacemaker generator model recorded in room in which implantation is performed **Exception:** Temporary pacemaker	100
10. Type of electrode catheter recorded in room in which implantation is performed **Exception:** Temporary pacemaker	100
11. Report by operating surgeon on (a) preoperative diagnosis, (b) procedures performed, and (c) description of tissues and findings, dictated or written immediately after surgery	100
12. Management of complications	
a. Skin necrosis	
(1) Pacemaker repositioned	100
(2) Culture and sensitivity of skin lesion	100
(3) Antibiotic consistent with culture and sensitivity	100
b. Hematoma	
Aspiration of hematoma	100
c. Wound infection	
(1) Wound drained	100
(2) Culture and sensitivity of drainage	100
(3) Antibiotic consistent with culture and sensitivity	100
(4) In presence of gross infection, alternative pacing system implanted **Exception:** Infection readily controlled	100

Criterion	Standard (in %)
d. Pacemaker malfunction	
Pacemaker repositioned	100
e. Pacemaker failure	
Alternative pacing system implanted	100

POSTOPERATIVE CARE

13. Anesthetist's postoperative evaluation of patient following transfer from recovery room — 100
14. EKG monitoring
    a. Constantly for at least 2 days post-operatively — 100
    b. Thereafter, daily EKG until discharge — 100
15. Patient at complete bed rest on back or left side for 24 hours postoperatively — 100
16. Postoperative nursing care
    a. Vital signs every 15 minutes until stable, then in accordance with postoperative care plan — 100
    b. Intravenous therapy and medications monitored and maintained — 100
    c. Daily charting of patient's condition and progress — 100
    d. Patient monitored for evidence of complications — 100

LENGTH OF STAY

17. Length of stay 6 to 10 days — 100
    Exceptions: (a) Early departure against medical advice; (b) presence of complications or other diagnoses such as cerebral vascular disease, peripheral vascular disease, chronic congestive heart failure, or recent myocardial infarction justifying extension.

DISCHARGE STATUS

18. Patient discharged under the following conditions:

Criterion	Standard (in %)
a. Satisfactory functioning of pacemaker as reflected in EKG	100
b. Improvement in cardiac and general condition of patient	100
c. Patient and family instructed re (1) follow-up visit to physician, (2) any applicable dietary restrictions, (3) dosages and schedules of applicable medications, and (4) need to avoid electrical hazards, including proximity to microwave ovens	100
Exception: Instructions on transfer form	

Appendix 3

QUALITY ASSURANCE REVIEW REPORT

DEPARTMENT OR SERVICE _____

SUBJECT OF REPORT _____ DATE _____

TYPE OF REVIEW
  Routine periodic   _____
  Medical staff requirement   _____
  Profile data response   _____
    Utilization   _____
    Clinical performance   _____
    Morbidity screen   _____
  Incident data response   _____
  Other rationale for review   _____
    Specify:

STUDY SAMPLE (Size, composition, time frame, defining characteristics)

DATA SOURCES

REVIEW CRITERIA APPLIED

PRINCIPAL FINDINGS

ACTION PLANNED OR TAKEN
  Responsible agents:

  Target date for progress or final report on action:

FOLLOW-UP STUDY
  Not necessary _____
  Target date for follow-up study:

DATA RETRIEVAL TECHNIQUES USED (Please circle all used)
  Concurrent monitoring
  Retrospective review
  Combination
FINDINGS REPORTED TO

Appendix 4

GANTT LAYOUT CHART

Project: Developing and Implementing a Rubella Control Policy

Task	July 1984 6 13 20 27	August 1984 3 10 17 24 31	Sept. 1984 7 14 21 28
1. Initial research including Determine Health Department requirements Survey all area hospitals for their policies Submit tables showing survey results to Infection Control Committee for review			
2. Draft proposed policy and procedure document for submission to Infection Control Committee			
3. Survey present personnel files for evidence of previous immunization			
4. Review and approval of proposed policy by Infection Control Committee and submission to administration and medical staff for final approval			
5. Orient the following to proposed policy: Personnel department All department heads Laboratories Accounting			
6. Prepare and print explanatory announcement for personnel			
7. Policy approved by administration and medical staff			
8. Distribute employee announcement			
9. Policy implemented with respect to new hires			

Appendix 5

CRITICAL PATH NETWORK

Project: Development and Implementation
of Rubella Control Policy

Tasks or activities:
   A.   Research area hospitals' rubella policies and prepare
        table
   B.   Draft rubella policy document
   C.   Review personnel records for previous immunization
   D.   Revise policy document for submission to administration
        and medical staff for approval
   E.   Orient personnel department, accounting department,
        and all department heads to new policy

Nodes or endpoints:
   1.   Start of project
   2.   Committee acceptance and review of survey findings
   3.   Committee acceptance and review of draft policy
        document
   4.   Acceptance, review, and approval of document by
        administration and medical staff
   5.   Beginning of implementation of policy and end of
        project

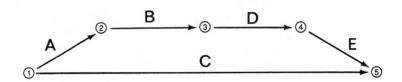

Appendix 6

QUALITY ASSURANCE PROGRAM
ANNUAL EVALUATION

Summary of Compliance with Hospital Criteria
1982–1983

	Percentage of Compliance		
Criterion	*1982*	*1983*	*Change (in %)*
Justified admissions	85	95	+10
Presence of indications for blood transfusion	75	85	+10
Absence of unjustified length of stay	60	75	+15
Absence of surgical wound infections	90	95	+ 5
Preadmission screening in elective surgery	55	75	+20
Third-party payer claims accepted as submitted	80	90	+10

Notes

1. L. Dunn, "Hospital Corporate Liability: The Trend Continues," *Medicolegal News*, October 1980, p. 16.

2. Ibid., p. 17.

3. E. Codman, Report. *Proceedings of the Philadelphia County Medical Society, 1913*.

4. J. Carroll and S. Becker, "On the Paucity of Course Work in Evaluation Research," *Journal of Medical Education*, January 1975, p. 38.

5. Unpublished survey by Jean Carroll Associates, September 1980.

6. R. Johnson, "Hospital Boards Should Abandon Medical Staff 'Self-Governance,'" *Modern Healthcare*, July 1983, pp. 134–40.

7. *JCAH Bulletin*, March 1953.

8. *JCAH Bulletin*, March 1955.

9. Accreditation Manual for Hospitals, 1984 (Chicago: Joint Commission on Accreditation of Hospitals, 1983), p. 149.

10. Unpublished interview material, June 1980.

Bibliography

American Hospital Association. Hospital Administrative Services Monitrend Reports. July 1982; December 1982; July 1983; December 1983.

_____. Hospital Statistics 1979, 1980, 1981, 1982, and 1983. Chicago: American Hospital Association.

Anderson, O., and M. Shields. "Quality Measurement and Control in Physician Decision Making: State of the Art." *Health Services Research,* Summer 1982, pp. 125–55.

Becker, S., and D. Neuhauser. *The Efficient Organization.* New York: Elsevier-North Holland Publishing, 1975.

Bertram, D. A. "Managing an Emergency Department: The Effect of Patient Flow on Physician Performance." *Quality Review Bulletin,* June 1983, p. 175.

Carroll, J. "Performance Appraisal in Medical Institutions." Report of the First Institute on Medical School Administration. Evanston, Ill.: Association of American Medical Colleges, 1964.

_____. "The Structure of Teaching Hospitals." Proceedings of the Twenty First Annual Meeting of the Association of University Programs in Hospital Administration. Chicago: Association of University Programs in Hospital Administration, 1969.

_____. Patient Care Audit Criteria. Homewood, Ill.: Dow Jones-Irwin, 1983.

Carroll, J., and S. Becker. "On the Paucity of Course Work in Evaluation Research." *Journal of Medical Education,* January 1975.

Cochran, W. G. *Sampling Techniques.* New York: John Wiley & Sons, 1964.

Codman, E. Report in Proceedings of the Philadelphia County Medical Society. 1913.

Dunn, L. "Hospital Corporate Liability: The Trend Continues." *Medicolegal News,* October 1980, pp. 16–29.

Ewell, C. "Trends May Intensify MD–CEO Tensions." *Modern Healthcare,* September 1983, pp. 210–11.

Flanagan, J. B., and K. J. Sourapas. "Preparing for Prospective Payment." *Journal of the American Medical Record Association,* February 1984, pp. 15–17.

Hughes, K., H. Dalsey, and W. Patterson. "Predicting Acute Care Hospital Bed Need through Physician Inpatient Activity Modeling: First Steps." *Health Care Strategic Management,* October 1983, pp. 8–11.

Johnson, Richard. "Hospital Boards Should Abandon Medical Staff 'Self-Governance'." *Modern Healthcare,* July 1983, pp. 134–40.

Joint Commission on Accreditation of Hospitals. Accreditation Manual for Hospitals, 1970, 1974, 1975, 1983. Chicago: Joint Commission on Accreditation of Hospitals.

_____. *JCAH Bulletin,* November 1952.

_____. *JCAH Bulletin,* March 1953.

_____. *JCAH Bulletin,* August 1953.

_____. *JCAH Bulletin,* March 1954.

_____. *JCAH Bulletin,* May 1954.

_____. *JCAH Perspectives,* January–February 1984.

Kaufman, K. "Deregulation of the Health Care Industry: Implications of Financial Change." *Health Care Strategic Management,* October 1983, pp. 4–7.

Keegan, A. "Scared Hospitals Cower." *Modern Healthcare,* November 1983, p. 160.

Knaus, W. A.; E. A. Draper; and D. P. Wagner. "Toward Quality Review in Intensive Care: The APACHE System." *Quality Review Bulletin,* July 1983, p. 196.

Kraft, J. G. "Preferred Provider Organizations: Addressing the Legal Issues." *Healthcare Financial Management,* August 1983, pp. 10–16.

Leavitt, T. "Marketing Success Through Differentiation—of Anything." *Harvard Business Review,* January–February 1980, pp. 83–91.

Lindner, J., and D. Wagner. "DRGs Spur Management-Related Groups." *Modern Healthcare,* May 1983, pp. 160–61.

March, J., and H. Simon. *Organizations.* New York: John Wiley & Sons, 1958.

Neubauer-Rice, R. "Preparing for the DRG-Based Prospective Rate System." *Quality Review Bulletin,* August 1983, p. 236.

Orifice, J. J., and M. Jennings. "Productivity—A Key to Managing Cost per Case." *Healthcare Financial Management,* August 1983, pp. 18–24.

Punch, L. "Emergicenters Serve HMO Enrollees." *Modern Healthcare,* October 1983, p. 32.

Sandrick, K. M. "Cost Containment: Blue Cross-Blue Shield's PROBE Information Reporting System." *Quality Review Bulletin,* September 1983, p. 272.

————. "Cost Containment: The GAO's Report on Educating Physicians in Cost Containment Issues." *Quality Review Bulletin.* February 1983, p. 36.

Schacter, M., G. Oppenheimer, L. Cannoodt, and S. Sieverts. "Evaluation of a Surgical Second Opinion Program." *Quality Review Bulletin,* January 1983, p. 11.

Schlicke, C. P. "American Surgery's Noblest Experiment." *Journal of the American Medical Association,* January 1973.

Serluco, R. J., and K. Johnson. "Cost Containment: Importance of the Medical Record Process in a DRG Based System." *Quality Review Bulletin,* September 1983, p. 268.

Siegel, S. *Nonparametric Statistics for the Behavioral Sciences.* New York: McGraw-Hill, 1956.

Snedecor, G. W. *Statistical Methods.* Ames, Ia.: Iowa State University Press, 1970.

Spirer, H. *Business Statistics: A Problem-Solving Approach.* Homewood, Ill.: Dow Jones-Irwin, 1975.

Stern, A. "Instilling Activism in Trustees." *Harvard Business Review,* January–February 1980, pp. 24–32.

Studnicki, J., and D. Honemann. "Analyzing Inpatient Hospital Duration and Intensity, Part II." *Quality Review Bulletin,* May 1983, p. 139.

U.S. Department of Commerce. *Statistical Abstract of the United States, 1982–1983.* Washington, D.C.: U.S. Government Printing Office, 1984.

Young, D. W. "Medical Practice, Case Mix, and Cost Containment." *Journal of the American Medical Record Association,* February 1982, pp. 801–5.

Zelman, W. N., and W. F. Jessee. "Budgeting Quality Assurance Activities." *Quality Review Bulletin,* February 1983, p. 42.

Index